SCRAWNY
TO
BRAWNY

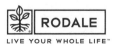
RODALE
LIVE YOUR WHOLE LIFE™

Every day our brands connect with and inspire millions of people to live a life of the mind, body, spirit — a whole life.

SCRAWNY TO BRAWNY

MICHAEL MEJIA   JOHN BERARDI

THE COMPLETE GUIDE TO BUILDING MUSCLE THE NATURAL WAY

RODALE

© 2005 by Michael Mejia and John Berardi
Photographs © 2005 by Rodale Inc.

Printed in the United States of America
Rodale Inc. makes every effort to use acid-free ♾, recycled paper ♻.

Book design by Susan P. Eugster
Photographs by Mitch Mandel
Illustrations by Karen Kuchar

Library of Congress Cataloging-in-Publication Data

Mejia, Michael.
      Scrawny to brawny : the complete guide to building muscle the natural way / Michael Mejia
and John Berardi.
            p.   cm.
      Includes index.
      ISBN-13 978–1–59486–088–1 paperback
      ISBN-10 1–59486–088–2 paperback
      1. Bodybuilding—Handbooks, manuals, etc.   2. Bodybuilders—Nutrition.   3. Muscle
strength.   I. Berardi, John.   II. Title.
      GV546.5.M44   2005
      613.7'13—dc22   2004027349

Distributed to the trade by Holtzbrinck Publishers

8   10   9   7   paperback

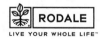

LIVE YOUR WHOLE LIFE™

We inspire and enable people to improve their lives and the world around them
For more of our products visit **rodalestore.com** or call 1-800-848-4735

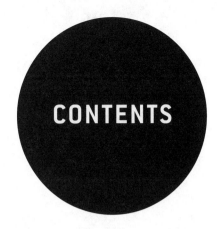

CONTENTS

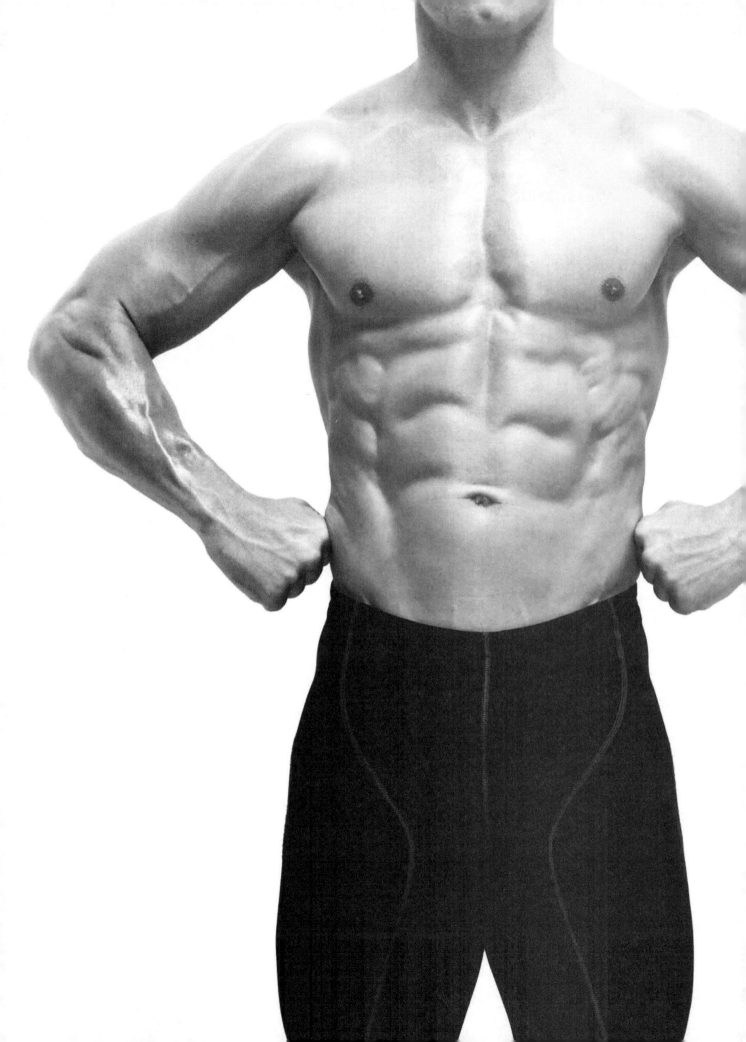

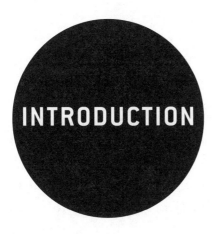

INTRODUCTION

FRUSTRATIONS OF A LIFELONG "HARDGAINER"

》》Hey, Skinny! Yeah, I'm talking to you. Or maybe you prefer String Bean, or Gumby, or how about Bones? What? Like you've never been called at least one of these about a dozen times before. Every time you don a T-shirt, wear shorts on a hot day, or worst of all, go shirtless at the beach, you immediately become an object of ridicule. You're pitied by women and mocked by guys with I.Q. scores only slightly surpassing the circumference of their biceps.

But hey, maybe none of that bothers you. Maybe you're the type who's content to let other guys lug around all those pesky muscles; you know, the kind that your significant other just drools over. Or maybe you've just convinced yourself to accept these "perks" because the truth is just too damn painful.

The truth is you're tired of busting your hump in the gym and not seeing any results. You're fed up with working twice as hard as the guy on the bench next to you who seems to grow like a weed while all you can manage to do is resemble one. You're sick of all the pills, powders, and shakes that promise the physique of your dreams but deliver nothing but gastrointestinal distress. But mostly you've just had it with all the wisecracks and putdowns you have to endure on a daily basis.

In fact, the only thing worse is listening to all the half-baked advice you get from friends, family, and fellow gymgoers who pretend to understand your plight. Things like "You've got to eat more." Really. Or, "You gotta train harder." I see, so inducing an aneurysm is the goal then? Or, my personal favorite: "You're wasting your time; guys like you just can't get big." ARRRGGGHHHHHH!

If I sound like I speak from experience, it's because I do. You see, like you, I too was once a "skinny guy." Born with the classic long limbs and short muscle bellies that typify an ectomorphic physique (more on this distinction later), I never realized the disadvantages I would later face when discovering my penchant for pumping iron. You see, long arms and legs mean that weights have to travel an awful long way when being lifted. But we'll get to that soon enough. Besides, it wasn't all bad; having the wingspan of a condor came in rather handy as a kid on the playground. It made me a natural at blocking shots and snagging rebounds on the basketball court. And don't even get me started on throwing sports. Whether it was a baseball or a football, those same long limbs I would later come to curse allowed me to sport an absolute cannon for arm. Yeah, I guess you could say that despite a glaringly obvious lack of anything that even closely resembled speed, I was your basic 16-year-old athletic prodigy.

Unfortunately, raw natural ability can take you only so far. So, seeing as how there weren't too many 6'1", 160-pound quarterbacks in the NFL, I figured I was going to need a big-time body to go along with my big-time arm. This realization prompted my very first foray into the weight room. It was there, in my friend's basement as a 16-year-old neophyte, where I first learned just what a cruel genetic trick my parents had played on me. Training beside guys whose muscles seemed to inflate at the mere sight of a loaded barbell, I spent the most grueling and fruitless summer of my life.

Despite the fact that I trained harder and more diligently than anyone else, I had the least results to show for my efforts. In fact, it got so bad that, no longer wanting to be bothered with the chore of loading and unloading the bar between sets, my friend suggested that I work out on the other bench with his little brother. It was the weight room equivalent of being banished to the Thanksgiving kiddie table and it was absolutely humiliating.

I must admit, though, that it did prepare me for what I was about to endure for the next several years. Undaunted by my inability to gain any appre-

ciable amount of muscle mass, I continued to hit the weights all through high school, even after my playing days were long since over. In fact, it became such an obsession that by the time I was 19, I was working as an instructor at a local health club, and by 21 I was working my way through college as a personal trainer—a successful one, I might add. Ironic, isn't it? Here I was, unable to reach my own physical goals, and yet I became rather adept at helping my growing clientele reach theirs. Talk about frustrating! Not to mention, pretty embarrassing.

I mean, come on, you'd think that someone in my position would have a decided advantage when it came to building up his body. After all, I was in the gym constantly, knew tons about exercise and nutrition, and had the responsibility of feeling I had to "look the part" driving me. The funny thing is, in retrospect, I'd have to say that these factors actually wound up working against me. That's right: All that time in the gym and all those hours I spent reading about and experimenting with different workouts turned out to be somewhat of a liability. Oh sure, I learned a lot. Trouble is, the more I learned, the more scientific I became in my approach to training. And the more scientific I became, the more I drifted away from the heavy, basic lifts my body needed to grow.

Thus began the period of my training career that I jokingly refer to as the lost decade. During that time I tried almost every program known to man: fast reps, slow reps, high reps, low reps (wasn't that a Dr. Seuss book?) with little if anything to show for it. Not to mention spending the equivalent of the GNP on supplements. And still nothing! Don't get me wrong; I was in shape, but if you looked at me, you'd never guess that I lifted as seriously as I did. I used to get asked all the time if I was a runner or a swimmer or where I left my horse Pokey. And those were the polite comments; I won't even go into the stuff I used to hear from the meatheads in the weight room when I dared to bring my clients in there. Yep, it was a tough time, all right.

Fast forward to the mid-90s. I was in a bookstore perusing the exercise titles when I came across a book geared toward "hardgainers." Having never heard this term before, I was intrigued and decided to give it a look. After all, I certainly had a hard enough time gaining muscle. Inside it talked about some people's difficulty in putting on muscle mass with the conventional approach to training. It recommended less frequent, but more intense workouts with far less volume than I was used to as a means of maximizing recovery between training sessions. It talked about the importance of basic, heavy lifts, highlighting the fact that isolation movements were of limited value to some lifters. In short, it was exactly what I had been looking for.

In the beginning, my results were good. I started lifting heavier weights and my body really seemed to be responding to all the extra recovery time between workouts. I started to gain a little bit of weight and actually looked somewhat bigger. Unfortunately, my euphoria was short-lived, as several little problems started to surface a few months into the program. I quickly learned why I hadn't been doing a lot of benching and squatting prior to this point. Because I sucked at them! As I alluded to earlier, when you have arms like an orangutan and legs like a giraffe, the bar has to travel an awful long way. This made attempting to increase the poundage on these lifts rather frustrating—not to mention the fact that the workouts, though intense, were somewhat monotonous.

Gone was all the variety of my previous workouts. I went from super setting three different exercises for my chest to inching up my bench each week. And I pretty much eliminated isolation exercises like leg extensions and lateral raises in favor of squats and overhead presses. True, I did gain some muscle, but my results were somewhat imbalanced, to say the least. It seemed that all the emphasis on chest and lat work was creating a rather noticeable round-shouldered slump to my posture. All the squatting and deadlifting was placing far too much emphasis on my glutes, causing them to become overdeveloped in relation to the rest of my body. It created a rather interesting visual effect. I went from looking like a swizzle stick, to a somewhat larger swizzle stick with poor posture and a huge butt.

I decided to abandon the hardgainer approach for a while and go back to my old style of training. All the while, though, I was consumed with thinking of ways I could somehow alter the program so that I could still make gains, without throwing my body completely out of whack. Coincidentally, this was taking place right around the time I was set to attend a training and nutrition conference where my coauthor, John Berardi, would be presenting. Although I hadn't met him at the time, I had heard of John and was looking forward to his reportedly innovative views on performance nutrition. My interest was especially piqued when I found out he'd be doing a presentation on eating to gain muscle mass.

John began his presentation with a statement that immediately got my attention. "The average guy trains hard enough to grow but doesn't eat anywhere near enough to support that growth." Granted, it wasn't anything earth-shattering; plenty of people had told me that I needed to eat more if I wanted to gain size. The difference was that John had developed formulas for calculating caloric requirements that far exceeded the recommended norms at that time. For instance, according to John's formula, I was taking in more than 1,000 calories per day fewer than I needed to support muscle gain! And here I was thinking that I was consuming a 500-calorie-per-day surplus based on the more traditional formula I had used to calculate my daily energy needs. He also presented some extremely interesting data on how he strategically combined specific macronutrients at certain times to help his clients successfully gain substantial amounts of muscle mass.

That was it; I was sold. I thought to myself, if this guy can produce these kinds of results and he's built like an ox himself, he must know what he's talking about. So, armed with the information John presented in his lecture and an even stronger resolve to fix my perceived shortcomings with the traditional hardgainer approach, I returned to the gym on an absolute mission. I didn't care what it took (well, I wasn't about to start doing steroids, but serious training and nutrition were fair game); I wasn't going to be stopped until I put on some size. And lo and behold, three months later I had gained 10 pounds of solid muscle. Now that may not seem like much to some, but to someone who hadn't put on 10 pounds after a decade of hard training, it was positively exhilarating. My legs looked thicker, my shoulders broader, and I was actually putting some strain on my shirtsleeves. For the first time in my life, I looked like I lifted weights. It felt fantastic!

Not that aesthetics was the only thing that mattered to me—my primary concern was and always has been achieving a good standard of physical health. But when you've spent as much time as I have in the weight room, you want to have a little something to show for it. Saying that I was satisfied with my lack of visible results after years of arduous training is a little like saying that I read *Playboy* just for the articles. While I may value and appreciate their editorial tone, it ain't exactly my reason for buying the magazine. So, while some may find it shallow, I must admit my new physique had me feeling pretty good. It improved my self-esteem somewhat and gave me the confidence to dispense training advice with greater authority. But more important, it made me want to tell anyone who would listen what finally worked after years of frustration.

One of the things that worked was eating like a bulimic Sumo wrestler. Okay, I'm partly kidding here. However, thanks to John Berardi, I learned that to get big, you have to eat big. And I'm not just talking some of the time. If you have a problem putting on muscle mass and you want to get bigger, you've got to eat constantly. You have to calculate the number of calories your body needs to support muscle growth and do whatever it takes to make sure you meet that number. There's no missing meals, no forgetting to eat; you have to arm yourself with a constant supply of healthy snacks and always make sure you have access to the kinds of foods you need to get in all the proper nutrients. Any failure to meet these energy requirements will render even the most well-designed program practically useless. Trust me on this one.

The other thing that worked was combining the simplicity of the original hardgainer approach with some of the more scientific training principles I had learned earlier in my career. For instance, by simply tweaking the way basic, staple lifts like squats, dead lifts, and bench presses were performed, I was able to place more emphasis on the muscle groups I was targeting and reduce the strain on joints and connective tissue. More important, though, the alterations I made, combined with a more balanced overall training approach, eliminated the muscle imbalances that had plagued my earlier attempts. The overdeveloped glutes and round-shouldered slump were replaced with more muscular thighs and dramatically improved upper back development. And, not coincidentally, I also experienced a noticeable decrease in those nagging little injuries that had always seemed to sabotage my progress.

Not content to revel in my own success, I started thinking of ways to spread the word about the training system I had developed. Or at least the one I had revamped, with the aid of one of the best nutritional minds in the business. After all, guys who needed this type of advice certainly weren't getting it from the mainstream media. If you're overweight in America today, you have a seemingly endless stream of resources at your disposal: books, diets, self-appointed weight loss gurus with their own talk shows who profess to have the solution to all of your problems. But if you're one of those rare few who's actually trying to *gain* weight, you're out of luck. For some strange reason, there's no shortage of compassion for the overweight, but tell people you're trying to pack on a few pounds, and they don't want to hear it.

Of course, there's always the muscle mags. Trouble is, all you're going to find there are ridiculously high-volume training programs that are best suited to either drug-enhanced lifters or the genetically gifted. There's no way the average drug-free trainee is going to make any substantial gains with these types of bodybuilding-inspired, "split" routines. And, if said lifter just happens to be an "ectomorph," he's really out of luck. As you'll soon come to discover, the majority of training information currently available to this segment of the population is completely inappropriate for their body type. Not to mention the fact that what little there is that does take into consideration their inherent physical differences is usually extremely generic.

You see, unlike other guys who seemingly blow up as soon as they pick up a weight, guys like you and me are different . . . *genetically* different. Not that I'm trying to play the genetics card as an excuse; I'm living proof that you can achieve substantial results when armed with the right information and a dogged determination to improve. I'm merely saying that it's a physiological fact that certain body types have a more difficult time gaining muscle mass. Like it or not, skinny guys in the weight room have to play by a different set of rules—rules you need to become intimately familiar with to obtain the kind of results you so desperately seek.

But don't worry; you've come to the right place. Because whether you're scrawny, you know someone who's scrawny, or you train people who are scrawny, the information contained in this book will produce results beyond what you ever imagined possible. It doesn't matter if you're a seasoned gym rat or an awkward teen who's getting his first exposure to strength training, follow our advice and gains of 10, 15, even up to 20 pounds aren't out of the question in as little as 16 weeks of training. You can pack on a few pounds of muscle or completely overhaul your physique; the choice is yours. It really all boils down to what you're looking to do and how well you stick to the plan.

How can I be so sure you'll make such impressive gains when everything else you've ever tried has failed? My certainty comes from the fact that I know exactly what you're going through. I've been called all the nicknames and gotten those same looks. The only difference between you and me is that I was in a position to do something about it. I did all the necessary research and sought out the best nutritional advice available. I even used myself and some of my hypertrophy-challenged clients as human guinea pigs to field-test my findings. And now I'm sharing it all with you. You get to be the beneficiary of all those years of backbreaking work and intensive study. My pain becomes your progress; my knowledge, your ultimate weapon in building the physique of your dreams.

No more gimmicks. No more false promises. From here on in, it's all about results—proven results from someone who knows what it is like to be in your shoes. And not only do I give you the information contained in this book—at www.scrawnytobrawny.com, you'll be able to commune with other individuals on the program, people facing the same challenges you are, supporting you every step of the way.

So, what are you waiting for? Come on, Skinny. We've got some work to do. ●

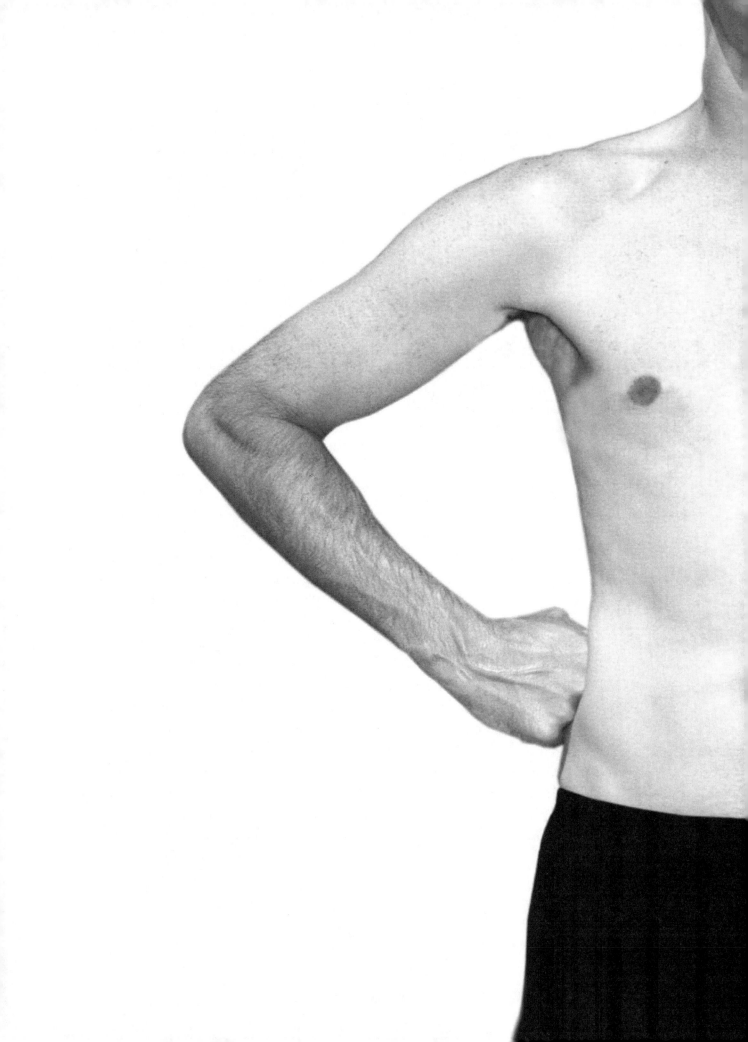

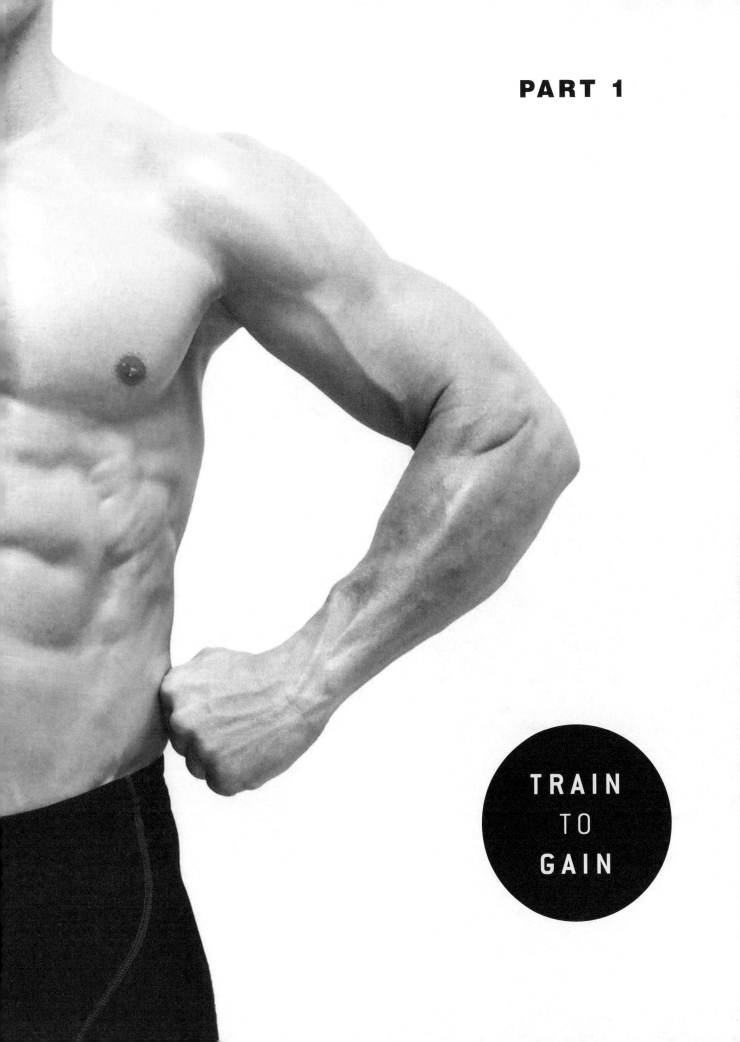

PART 1

TRAIN
TO
GAIN

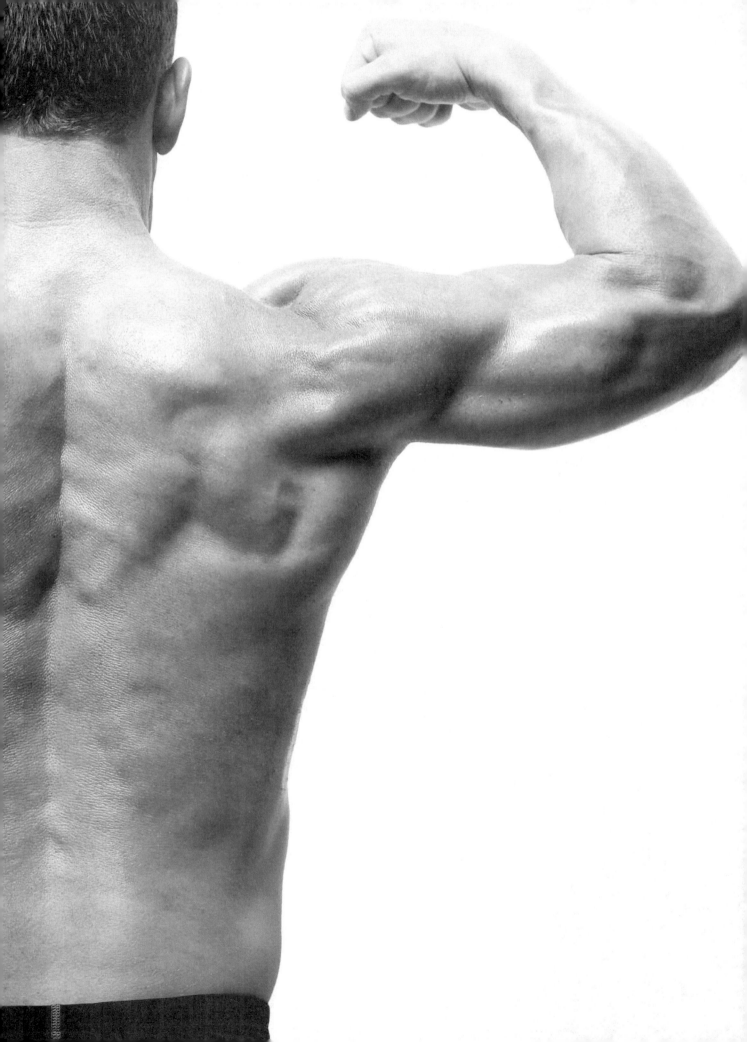

THE SKINNY ON
HARDGAINER TERMINOLOGY

Before we really start to get the ball rolling, the first thing we should do is define a couple of terms. Let's start with the three terms that popped up in the introduction, terms that you can bet your bottom dollar you'll see again. These terms are hypertrophy, ectomorph, and hardgainer. Let's start with hypertrophy. Hypertrophy is just a fancy way of speaking of muscle growth. So if we call you hypertrophy-challenged, that is simply our politically correct way of saying that you have a tough time building muscle.

Next, let's discuss ectomorph and hardgainer. Contrary to popular belief, these two terms are not interchangeable. The term ectomorph refers to a particular somatotype: a method for classifying different body types based on specific physical characteristics. The word hardgainer, on the other hand, is a contrived term that's used in the iron game to describe someone who has a difficult time gaining muscle mass. Because of their inability to make progress with more conventional training methods, most ectomorphs just automatically assume that they're hardgainers. When in truth, the very notion of even being a hardgainer is as fabricated as the term itself.

We realize that last statement comes as a bit of a shock. Not only does it fly in the face of just about everything you've ever been told about your inability to make appreciable gains in size and strength, but it also robs you of the best excuse you ever had. After all, it's much easier to throw around some cool-sounding gym lingo than it is to admit that you have no clue how to eat or train properly to reach your goals. Ouch, that had to hurt! But before we shatter your belief system by debunking this whole hardgainer myth, it might help to provide you with some insight into how the idea of body typing came to be in the first place and whether or not it actually holds any merit. At the very least, it will help you gain an understanding about why people respond differently to various forms of diet and exercise.

ENDOS AND MESOS AND ECTOS, OH MY!

There are three different somatotypes commonly used to classify the human body: endomorphs, mesomorphs, and ectomorphs (see below). Not that it's really that cut-and-dry; few people fit neatly into one specific category. Most of us exhibit characteristics of more than one somatotype at once. This somewhat crude form of genetic stereotyping is the brainchild of a psychologist by the name of William H. Sheldon, M.D. Back in the early 1940s, seeking to draw connections between body type and temperament, Sheldon studied the photographs of more than 4,000 college-age men. Based on his findings, he actually identified several different body types but later consolidated them, reasoning that everyone could be classified as some combination of the three we still use today.

Using a numerical system as a means of quanti-fying how much of each somatotype a person displayed, Sheldon introduced a unique three-digit code. Setting an order of endomorph, mesomorph, and ectomorph, Sheldon used a scale of 1 to 7 (the closer the number to 1, the less relation to the somatotype; the closer to 7, the greater) to assign values to each. So, for example, a true endomorph would be assigned a number of 711, a mesomorph 171, and an ectomorph 117. And no, 007 was not James Bond's somatotype; it was his agent number. Of course, since few people fit into one specific mold, numbers such as 541 (a combination endomorph and mesomorph), 246 (a combination ectomorph and mesomorph), and 153 (a combination mesomorph and ectomorph) are much more common.

As you might imagine, Sheldon's findings were widely criticized, mainly because he based his assertions solely on visual inspection of photographs

WHAT'S YOUR TYPE?

ECTOMORPHS: The typical ectomorph is a person who exhibits low levels of strength and size prior to training. They're usually tall and thin, with relatively low levels of body fat and small, narrow bones. Although their smaller joint structure often serves as an impediment in strength and power sports, they do tend to excel in endurance activities due to what is typically a higher-than-average proportion of slow twitch muscle fibers. Their fast metabolisms often make it difficult to gain weight of any type when following a more conventional dietary approach. Sheldon classified ectomorphs as being introverted, socially anxious individuals who tend to excel at mental tasks.

ENDOMORPHS: The endomorphic body type is considered to be the least desirable of the three major body types. Although endomorphs do tend to exhibit impressive levels of size and strength through training, they have a difficult time shedding body fat and gain weight rather easily. Sheldon believed endomorphs to be more focused on food and pleasure than physical activity. According to Sheldon, endomorphs typically have more jovial, easygoing personalities.

MESOMORPHS: These are the oft-referred-to genetically gifted individuals. They tend to exhibit low levels of body fat and impressive muscular development even prior to training. Their thick, wide bone structure is more conducive to building muscle, giving them a decided advantage in strength and power sports such as football, wrestling, and Olympic lifting. According to Sheldon, most mesomorphs are outgoing, adventurous individuals with action-oriented mentalities.

without any hard physiological data to back them up. Many other scientists argued that a person's body-type score shouldn't be based on something as easily altered as appearance. After all, would dropping 50 pounds change someone from an endomorph to an ectomorph? In Sheldon's system, probably. Therefore, researchers were interested in linking body type to some unchangeable physical features. Otherwise, as indicated, a poorly fed endomorph could wind up being classified as an ectomorph after losing a whack of body mass sweatin' to the oldies with Richard Simmons.

With Sheldon's system showing real weaknesses, two anthropometrists (that's a fancy term for a scientist who studies body measurements and dimensions), J. E. Lindsay Carter and Barbara Heath (1990) came up with a more scientific system for determining somatotypes. In their system, a skinfold-thickness measure was used to determine the degree of endomorphy; a height/weight ratio (termed the ponderal index) was used to measure ectomorphy; and the measurement of elbow joint and knee joint width as well as arm and calf circumferences was used to determine mesomorphy.

Carter and Heath's system was a good attempt but still a bit off the mark. True, they did attempt to link body type to actual anatomical characteristics. But, as with Sheldon's system, some of their choices were also *changeable* characteristics. Okay, maybe not height, but changing one's weight in relation to his height would certainly alter the ponderal index, just as it would alter skinfold thickness. So, although somewhat more objective, Carter and Heath's system was still essentially flawed. In our humble opinions, they should have turned their attention to something that was more finite, such as bone structure. Unlike muscle and fat mass, the overall dimensions of a person's bone structure don't change much once they've reached maturity.

NO BONES ABOUT IT

The ironic thing is that when using skeletal features as a means to assess body type, some of Sheldon's subjective assessments actually correlate rather well. For instance, Sheldon identified ectomorphs as being tall and thin with long limbs, mesomorphs as being broad-shouldered, and endomorphs as having a softer, rounder base. When comparing these descriptions with the skeletal method, we see that ectomorphs are represented by a more rectangular shape. Rectangles tend to be tall and thin, just like ectomorphs with their narrow shoulders and hips. Mesomorphs are depicted as inverted trapezoids. Inverted trapezoids are wider at the top and narrower toward the bottom, just like mesomorphs with their broad shoulders and narrow waists. Endomorphs exhibit a more classic trapezoid shape as a result of their wider bases. While very few male physiques tend to have the classic trapezoid shape of the endomorphic distinction, many men do carry a shape described best as mesendomorphic, characterized by wide hips *and* shoulders.

While we've been getting pretty technical in this section, the important thing to realize is that regardless of where you lie on this somatotypic, geometric continuum, few people can be pigeonholed into one specific somatotype. While you might be tall and thin, thus appearing to be a classic ectomorph, hiding under those medium T-shirts might be the potential of a godly physique. However, all this potential muscle will remain hidden if you fail to eat enough calories to support muscle growth and/or if you train in a manner contradictory to your goals. So don't immediately scream ectomorph, or worse yet, hardgainer. Too many people constantly use body type as a convenient excuse for their current physical status. Sure, it's a factor, but it's not the physiological scapegoat many make it out to be.

It's also worth noting that many of the telltale signs of a particular somatotype vary in degree from

(*continued on page 9*)

5

Believe it or not, labeling yourself an ectomorph isn't as simple as seeing if your fingertips touch when they encircle your wrist. Nor is it enough for you hypertrophy-challenged types to claim that you've "always been thin." Truth be told, there are a lot of potential mesomorphs hiding in skinny bodies. John, for example, went from a scrawny 160-pound guy to a brawny 210 pounds in just 2 years. By the same token, there are probably just as many endomorphs hiding in youthful, skinny bodies. Take a look at some of those skinny guys (who just assumed they were fat-gain-resistant ectomorphs by nature) about 10 years after graduation. They can't still think they're ectomorphs now, can they? These examples should make it clear that there are other factors besides "skinniness" that dictate someone's somatotype as well as their muscle-building potential.

Things such as the relationship between your shoulder and hip breadth, or the length of your femurs (thigh bones) in relation to your torso, are far more indicative of your inherent physical structure. Only when these are combined with information about your predominant muscle-fiber type can you begin to classify yourself with any degree of certainty. Although it should also be noted that hormonal factors come into play here as well, we'll spend more time discussing these factors in Chapter 4. The bottom line is that no one measure will tell you all you need to know about how your body will respond to training. The following measurements, though, should give you some valuable insights into what you'll ultimately be able to achieve. If you're curious about how you measure up, record the following, asking a friend to help as needed:

1. Height

2. Torso length: Measured from the acromion process (bony and prominent area at the top of the shoulder), to the top of the iliac crest (bony and prominent area at the top of the hip).

3. Femur length: Measured as the distance from the greater trochanter (bony and prominent area on the outside of your leg a couple of inches beneath your hip) and the lateral condyle of the knee (bony and prominent area on the outside of the knee).

4. Tibial (lower leg) length: Measured as the distance between the medial condyle (bony and prominent area on the inside of the knee) and medial malleolous of the

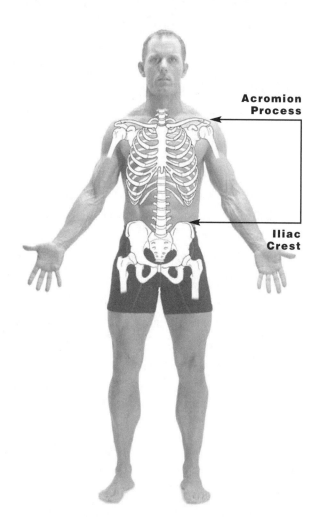

Acromion Process

Iliac Crest

TORSO LENGTH

tibia (bony and prominent area on the inside of the ankle).

5. Bi-acromial breadth: Measured as the distance between the acromion processes on each shoulder (bony and prominent areas at the top of each shoulder).

6. Bi-iliac breadth: Measured as the distance between the iliac crests of each hip (bony and prominent area at the top of the hip).

WHAT IT ALL MEANS

The shoulder to hip ratio: Take the bi-acromial distance, and divide it by the bi-iliac breadth. The larger this ratio, the more muscle mass you'll be able to carry on your frame. Values greater than 1.46 are optimal for building muscle mass.

The femur length to torso length relationship: A femur that's longer than your torso can compromise your ability to squat and deadlift efficiently because it will cause you to lean forward excessively to reach the desired depth. Of course, a femur and torso of near equal length combined with a shorter lower leg can sometimes pose similar problems, although this can often be effectively managed by improving flexibility around the ankle joint. For now, simply determining the relationship between these body segments to help identify where you might need additional flexibility work once you start the program.

(continued)

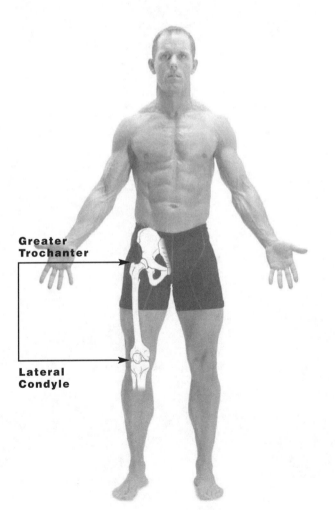

Greater Trochanter

Lateral Condyle

FEMUR LENGTH

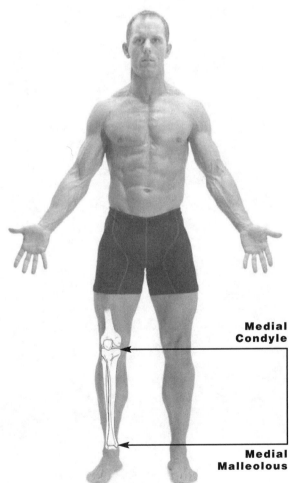

Medial Condyle

Medial Malleolous

TIBIAL LENGTH

MORPHOMETRICS: THE MEASURE OF A MAN—Continued

The shoulder width to height relationship: The larger the disparity between bi-acromial breadth and height, the more ectomorphic you are. So a 6'4" individual with a 14.5-inch bi-acromial breadth would be more ectomorphic than a 5'8" individual with the same size frame. Mike's shoulder width is 14.4" while his height is 73", giving him a shoulder width to height factor of 0.197. John's shoulder width is 14" while his height is 68", giving him a shoulder width to height factor of 0.206. As you can see from the previous discussion, Mike appears to be slightly more ectomorphic than John.

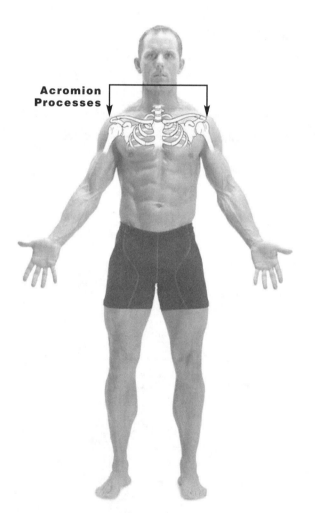

Acromion Processes

BI-ACROMIAL BREADTH

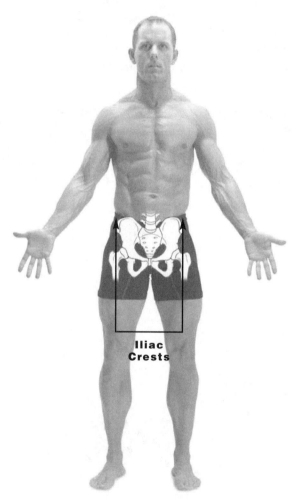

Iliac Crests

BI-ILIAC BREADTH

person to person. For instance, it's not uncommon to hear the assertion that many ectomorphs have long femurs (upper thigh bones) and short torsos. As you'll read in Chapter 3, this is something of a biomechanical albatross because it makes exercises such as squats and conventional deadlifts inordinately difficult. However, while certainly a hindrance, much of the added degree of difficulty in performing these lifts is dependent on just how much longer the femur is than the torso. A lifter whose femur is only slightly longer than his torso will have a much easier time than one who has a disparity of several inches. This is why things such as optimal depth on squats or how far to lower the bar during the bench press are individualized and depend greatly upon the relationship of various body segments.

In the end, the real value in taking these measures isn't to help you classify yourself as having a particular somatotype, but rather to give you an idea about how your individual anatomical structure affects the way you train. For instance, individuals with a bi-acromial to bi-iliac ratio of 1.46 or greater might attribute any difficulty in gaining muscle mass to suboptimal nutritional habits or overtraining, rather than any perceived degree of ectomorphy. This specific ratio, particularly when combined with more of a fast-twitch muscle fiber makeup (we show you how to assess this in the next chapter), has been associated with body-building success. Likewise if you have a torso, femur, and lower leg of near equal lengths, any difficulties you have in performing squats and deadlifts may be more due to flexibility issues than biomechanical considerations. However, even if you do come up with some undesirable numbers, the information contained in the following chapters can still help you level the playing field to a large degree.

The bottom line is that having a rough idea of

where your physical tendencies lie can save you a lot of time and effort that would have been otherwise wasted by training in a manner that wasn't suited to you. For instance, someone with strong ectomorphic tendencies isn't going to see the same kind of results as a more mesomorphic individual in following the high-volume training programs featured in most muscle mags. By the same token, a person who leans toward endomorphy and wants to drop a few pounds will likely have to do a lot more cardio work than a naturally lean person could get away with. This isn't just our opinion; it's a physiological fact that's verified on a daily basis in gyms nationwide by people who continue to toil away in frustration with nothing to show for their efforts. The sad part is that it doesn't have to be this way.

HARD TO SWALLOW

By now, our hypothesis should be clear. We believe that specific physical traits can and do dictate what a person needs to do from both a training and a dietary approach. After all, the major premise of this book is helping those of you who are hypertrophy-challenged put on some size, regardless of whether those challenges are real or perceived. We do, however, take issue with the position that a person's somatotype completely dictates his genetic potential. Granted, having specific physical characteristics may predispose you to success in a particular sport or activity, but it should by no means dissuade you from participating in others that you may not be best suited to.

If you need a few inspiring stories, look no further than the professional athletic realm. Professional sports have always been filled with athletes who excelled in spite of their physical "limitations." Take former NBA guards Spud Webb (5'7") and Mugsy Bogues (5'3"). These guys weren't exactly built for their sport, yet they excelled. Not to mention baseball god Babe Ruth—arguably the game's greatest player despite a physique more conducive to sitting at home rather than rounding toward it. And let's not forget former Mr. Olympia Frank Zane, who transformed his gangly, 98-pound body into one of the most aesthetically appealing physiques to ever grace a competitive stage.

The point is, you shouldn't listen to all the naysayers who tell you that it's impossible to overcome genetics. Although it's obvious that people with ectomorphic tendencies have a much harder time gaining muscle mass, it doesn't mean that they're doomed to a lifetime of physical frailty. If either of us had bought into that, we wouldn't have ever written this book in the first place. We would have remained two thin, unimposing (albeit terribly good-looking) unknowns. Instead, we chose to challenge conventional wisdom and come up with special solutions. In doing so, we formulated a plan of action that could be repeated. Now, this plan is available right here in this book. It serves as a template for others who share in what used to be our puny plight. By thinking outside the box and refusing to accept our genetic deficiencies, we've developed a system that will forever change the perception of what it means to be a skinny guy— more specifically, a skinny guy who pumps iron.

Now that we've got you all fired up, we'd better be frank. This is going to be a major undertaking. Many people out there, including various training "experts," liken the sight of a so-called ectomorph in the weight room to Al Sharpton running for president—nice thought and all, but a complete waste of time. No matter how hard they push themselves, they'll never really make it past a certain level of development or a certain number of constituents, whatever the case may be. And to a certain extent, they're right (sorry, Al). The key factor being that when you have a difficult time gaining size, it's not just about training hard; it's about training the right way. When you're cursed with traits such as long limbs and a Ferrari-like metabolism, you simply have to play by a different set of rules when it comes to strength training. You have to learn to train with greater intensity, less frequency, and much more dedication than the average lifter.

Once you come to terms with this simple fact, you'll begin to understand our disdain for the term hardgainer. Anyone would have trouble making gains when he's following a program that's completely inappropriate for his physical structure! Show us a tall, lanky lifter who spends the bulk of his time trying to up the poundage on his squat and bench press, and we'll show you one frustrated guy. Now, take that same lifter and give him *specific* dietary guidelines to follow, and he'll start growing. Then, tweak those same basic lifts (bench press, deadlift, squat) to accommodate for some of his biomechanical issues, and he'll literally start growing overnight. It's that simple. All it takes is some hard work and an open mind.

These days, it seems that anyone who can't get the results they're looking for immediately labels himself a hardgainer. Never mind the fact that his training program is designed for someone else's body and that his daily energy consumption wouldn't satisfy a hummingbird. The truth is that the majority of hardgainers are nothing of the sort. Overtrainers? Probably. Undereaters? Most definitely! But hardgainers? Sorry, we're just not buying it; particularly not in the case of you so-called ectomorphs, who, in our experience, almost always combine overtraining with a suboptimal caloric intake. It's impossible to get any bigger and stronger when you not only push your body beyond its capacity to recover but, on top of that, fail to provide it with enough of the nutrients it needs to repair itself.

C'mon, aren't you sick of making excuses? Isn't

it about time for a change? You wouldn't keep bringing your car to a mechanic who was never able to fix what was wrong with it. So why continue to stick with eating habits and workouts that don't deliver the kind of results you're looking for? Stop blaming your genetics, and start thinking outside the box. Regardless of what you've been led to believe, you *do* have the potential to develop impressive amounts of size and strength. Okay, so maybe you'll never win a bench press competition (Chapter 3 will explain why), but follow our program, and pretty soon your old max will be your new warmup. As long as you're willing to put in the work, both in the gym and the kitchen, we guarantee that you'll see significant improvement on all of your lifts. Want to hear something even more amazing? With this program, we plan to help you put some serious size on those stick-like arms of yours without so much as doing a single biceps curl!

Just do us a favor. Before we get started, drop the hardgainer tag. If you really feel the need to label yourself, from now on you're what's known as a lessimorph. It's a body type that responds best to brief, intense workouts (less is more—get it!) Seriously though, for convenience sake, from here on out, we're going to be referring to you as an ectomorph. Don't sweat it if you're not; there's still a ton of worthwhile training and nutritional information in the pages that follow for anyone who has a hard time gaining muscle mass. It's just that settling on a common term to identify our scrawny brethren is a lot easier than constantly referring to you as being "hypertrophy-challenged" or as having "ectomorphic tendencies." Not to mention the fact that it'll be a lot less annoying for all of us.

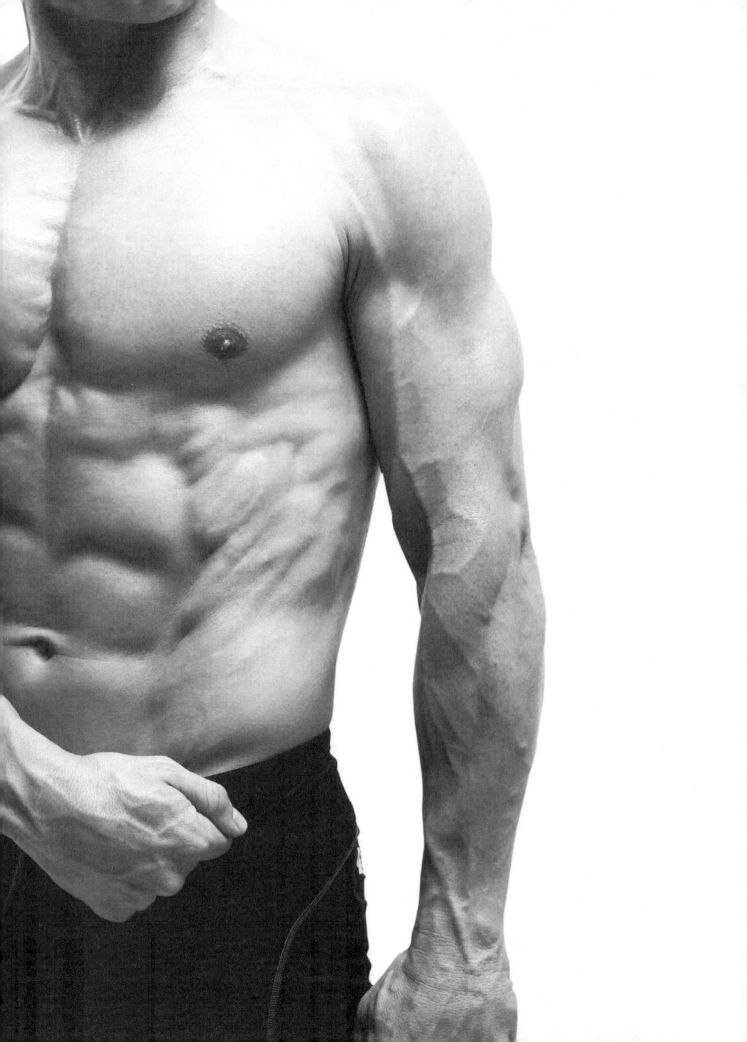

DIFFERENT STROKES
FOR SKINNY FOLKS

>> In the previous chapter, you should have taken some measurements and pinpointed some challenges that might come up in your quest for brawn. Based on the results of your measurements, you should now know if you've got scrawny-man tendencies. If it turns out that you do, don't sweat it. Okay, so maybe you don't muscle up as easily as most and have to work twice as hard for what little results you do get. You're also able to drop body fat at will, so the news isn't all bad. It's just a matter of coming to grips with the fact that the traditional approach to strength training doesn't work for you. Or better yet, taking the time to learn the hows and whys of exactly why it doesn't.

Simply put, conventional training programs don't get it done for ectomorphs. Unlike most guys, you can't just walk into gyms and begin lifting weights with the intention of "feeling the burn" and "working the muscles from different angles." Nope, body-building-style workout "splits" with different body-part pairings simply aren't going to cut it. Trying to get brawny this way is like trying to scrub a toilet with a toothbrush. Sure, it's funny, especially if it's not your toothbrush, but it's a complete waste of time and effort beyond the humor component. The minute you can begin to identify and appreciate your inherent physiological differences, the better you'll be at formulating strategies to overcome them.

And speaking of differences, there are four major factors working against the ectomorph in his quest for a more muscular physique. Here they are, in no particular order:

1. A muscle-fiber type better structured for endurance activity

2. Longer limb length

3. An accelerated metabolic rate

4. Long tendons, short muscles

Any one of these on its own can play a major role in determining how much muscle you'll eventually build. Let's face it, when you can eat like Rosie O'Donnell with a tapeworm and not gain an ounce, or it takes you forever to complete one stinkin' rep on the bench press, you're going to have a hard time building muscle. But before we really sink our teeth into these genetic differences and, more important, teach you how to overcome them, let's first examine what makes the conventional approach such a poor choice for you muscularly challenged types.

INEFFICIENCY EXPERTS

To be completely fair, the mainstream, body-building-style approach to strength training does work for some people. There are plenty of guys training this way and making impressive gains. You see, not everybody has to bust his butt with deadlifts and squats just to build a little muscle mass. Some guys blow up like ticks by sticking mainly with machines and isolation exercises. But it's been our experience that guys like these are the exception and not the rule.

Guys who grow easily by doing traditional bodybuilding-style workouts usually fall into one of the following three categories:

1. They built their bodies with hard, heavy training but can maintain it with less difficult workouts.

2. They are genetically gifted mesomorphs who grow even when they sneeze.

3. They are on steroids, and the anabolic power of the drugs makes up for their lack of gym savvy.

Whichever the case, they're *not* genetically challenged ectomorphs. If you're hypertrophy challenged and think you can increase size or strength to any

significant degree with this type of training, you've got another think coming.

Besides, even if traditional weight-lifting workouts can help some people get results, we're not so certain that this way of training makes much sense from a physiological standpoint. Rather, it's just a system based on tradition and heavily influenced by gym equipment manufacturers. Just like Chris Rock said in an old stand-up comedy routine: "Just because you can do it, doesn't make it a good freakin' idea."

So what's wrong with the typical workout? Well, let's look at what the average gym workout might look like. The average guy walks into the gym, and after a lame attempt to pick up the receptionist and a few herky-jerky movements he considers "stretches," he makes a beeline to the bench press. After some poor form pressing, it's on to a few other chest exercises—many of which are performed on machines (more on why this is a bad idea in a moment). After chest work, it's on to the arms. There, he'll spend the better part of the next 45 minutes admiring himself in the mirror, imitating the sound of a water buffalo in labor while attempting to lift more weight than he can handle (poor form again). Then it's on to a couple of sets of crunches through a microscopic range of motion and one last shot at the receptionist before he calls it a day. Our trainee then repeats this ritual (or one similar) the next day, only this time turning his attention to his back and shoulders. Then it's perhaps a day or two off before doing both workouts one more time heading into the weekend.

If you think this is a comical exaggeration, you're only partially right. This caricature isn't too far off the mark. Oh yes, and in case you were wondering, we didn't forget to include the leg work in the previously discussed routine. After all, most guys in the weight room avoid serious leg training like it's the plague (we don't really count riding the stationary bike or performing nothing but leg curls and leg presses as serious leg training). And even when leg work is included, we're certainly not fond of the quarter rep squat exercise a lot of trainees are so enamored with. Not familiar with this one? Perhaps you perform it? The quarter rep squat exercise is the one where you load up a barbell with more weight than you can handle and squat down about 6 inches or so. If this sounds like you, read on, and we'll help you troubleshoot your squatting form in Chapter 3.

So, steering back to the original question after our digression, the kind of compartmentalized approach to training that includes all this split-type training is of extremely limited value to guys who have a hard time putting on size. Dividing the body into different units and blasting away at said units with a barrage of exercises and sets performed at every possible angle simply doesn't offer enough of an overload to spur any serious growth. How can this be, you ask? After all, extreme local muscular fatigue accompanies this type of training, and that's gotta count for something, right? Well, it does, but only if you're more interested in getting sore and tired than getting big and strong.

Don't confuse training (and fatigue) with a training response. Bodybuilding-style training primarily stimulates one type of muscle fiber, and heavy, basic training stimulates another. To paraphrase famed muscle researcher William Kraemer, "some weightlifters can spend decades training but will never train their fast-twitch fibers. Since the fast-twitch muscle fibers are the ones that respond best to training, it's important to include both heavy, basic lifts and explosive lifts (i.e., Olympic lifts such as the clean and jerk, or snatch) with lighter loads to maximize their development." Seeing as how ectomorphs typically have a lower proportion of fast-twitch muscle fibers than most, if their goal is to get bigger and stronger, it only makes sense to make the most of what they've got by targeting these fibers in their training.

WRONG DIVISION

The point is, if you're an ectomorph, you've got to stop treating your body like a series of unrelated muscle groups, and start thinking of it as a single organism. Forget all this chest, shoulders, and triceps, legs, back, and biceps nonsense. If your goal is to get bigger, then the entire organism has to get bigger. The best way to achieve this is to focus on lifts that allow you to engage the largest amount of muscle mass possible. This essentially means that lifts such as squats, deadlifts, cleans, rows, military presses, pullups, bench presses, and dips are going to serve as the basis for most of your workouts. Sure, you'll periodically include some more isolated lifts such as biceps curls and rotator cuff work as a means of targeting weak links in your physique, but for the most part, it's going to be all compound lifts all the time.

A compound lift is simply one that works several different muscle groups all at the same time. This usually means that more than one joint is involved in the movement. A great example of this is the squat. The squat involves the hip joint, the knee joint, and the ankle joint, making it the king of the compound movements.

With that in mind, we'd like to give you an idea of what the typical gym schedule should be for the typical hypertrophy-challenged individual. Upon arrival at the front desk, be sure to avoid eye contact with the receptionist. Remember, you've got no shot, for now at least. Besides, you'll be too busy sipping the pre-workout carbohydrate/protein shake you'll learn how to concoct in Chapter 15. There'll be plenty of time for small talk later, say like 12 to 14 weeks later.

After warming up and thoroughly loosening the muscles that surround the hips, knees, ankles, core, and shoulders (see Mobility Sequence 1 in Chapter 6), make a beeline straight to the squat rack. If you see someone doing biceps curls, politely ask him to move to another location, so you can use the equipment for its intended purpose. After a few warmup sets in the squat rack, get ready to expend the bulk of your energy getting through a few grueling sets. Next, limp on over to the pullup station, and crank out a few sets of as many reps as you can muster. By all means, feel free to add extra weight if you can. And no, in case you're wondering, the lat pulldown isn't an acceptable alternative (see Alternative Medicine). In fact, whenever possible, always opt for free weights over machines. Free weights require balance and coordination. Also, because they involve the activation of more muscles to help stabilize the weight (i.e., prevent the weight from falling on your head or the heads of onlookers), they cause a greater release of those all-important, all-natural muscle-building hormones into your bloodstream. Besides, free weight exercises look cooler, and that always impresses receptionists.

From there, it's on to military presses, followed perhaps by some weighted situps. Finally, it's important to immediately pull a post-workout drink out of your gym bag, and start chugging. Think of this post-workout drink as your final exercise. Then, get out of there as quickly as possible, and don't even think of lifting again for at least a day or two. Your next workout will then center on the deadlift, bench press, some form of rowing, and perhaps some additional ab/core work.

We realize this isn't what you're used to, but you won't always have to train this way. Eventually, once you've built up enough size, you'll be able to train with greater frequency and variety.

But for now at least, compound, free-weight lifts such as these are the way to go. In case you're unfamiliar with how to perform some of these lifts or aren't sure how to put a program together, don't sweat it. We've provided you with an entire program complete with exercise descriptions in the training section of the book which begins on page 63.

C'mon, admit it. Right about now, you've got your head cocked to one side making that sound Scooby-Doo makes when he's confused. After all, that can't be all there is to the workouts, right? We can almost hear you saying things like "What, are they serious? Only *one* exercise for my chest?" Or maybe you're more the "what's all this squat and deadlift nonsense—don't they know those lifts are *dangerous*?" type of guy. Then of course there's the ever-popular "but how are my arms supposed to grow if there aren't any arm exercises?!?!?" There, there, everything's going to be okay. No need to get yourself so worked up. Stop reading for a second, and go into the kitchen to get a brown paper bag to help with the hyperventilating. It's all right; we'll wait. Good. Now, just take a few nice deep breaths, and we'll do our best to calm you back down.

IT AIN'T EASY BEING LEAN

All right, now that you're calm, we want to help unravel the confusion. Why don't most guys train as we're suggesting? Because it's hard. If it were easy, you'd see a heck of a lot more guys devoting the bulk of their training efforts to upping the poundage on their compound lifts. Instead, what you often see is set after set of mind-numbing isolation exercises. And who can blame them? It's a lot easier to do a set of lateral raises or leg extensions than a dizzying set of squats followed by a heavy, chest-heaving set of deadlifts. Some genetically gifted lifters have a choice. They can do either type of workout and see progress. Ectomorphs don't have this choice.

Feeling cheated? Well, trust us; we feel your pain. There were plenty of times when we were dying to start off our workout with a couple of sets of curls or by giving the really cool-looking new chest machine a whirl. Some days, these machines sure seem to beat the alternative—big squats in the power cage. But after years of not seeing the type of results we were looking for, we began to embrace the big squats and do them anyway. We're now urging you to do the same. As we said earlier, if you ever want to make any serious progress, you're going to have to learn to not only accept but also embrace your differences. The sooner you can come to terms with this simple fact, the sooner you'll start seeing results. Sure, it'll be tough; it takes a lot of discipline and self-confidence to swim against the tide of popular thinking. And it'll be even tougher still if you happen to train at home.

HOME ALONE

Yep, you read that last line correctly. Despite the numerous advantages associated with training in the privacy and comfort of your own home, there are, believe it or not, a couple of major drawbacks. Okay, so maybe you don't have to put up with smirks from a bunch of tank-top-clad gorillas who think a guy your size has no business near the free weights. But if you think it's tough starting your workout with squats in a climate-controlled gym, try it in a garage or basement at 5:00 A.M. on a cold winter's morning. Talk about dedication! Standing there next to a bag of fertilizer and your kid's bike, it's almost too tempting to scrap the heavy lifting protocol and settle in to some kinder, gentler isolation exercises. Besides, who would know? You could claim to train like a beast and just blame your genetics for your lack of progress.

Aside from having a built-in excuse, the other thing you have working against you is a relative dearth of appropriate training information at your disposal. As we mentioned earlier, the majority of fitness-related titles at your local Barnes & Noble deal with either weight loss or bodybuilding. And it's not like you can just open up a magazine or log on to a Web site and give the latest "can't miss" workout a try. Well, you can; you just probably won't like the results. That's because most workouts simply aren't designed with guys like you in mind. Things like your muscle fiber composition and limb length have labeled you in the minds of some as the fitness equivalent of a redheaded stepchild. Up until now, the best you could hope for is some generic training advice mixed in amidst the constant reminders that your lack of physical stature is more or less a genetic inevitability. Up until now, that is.

TAKING THE FOURTH

As any great military strategist will tell you, to defeat your enemy, you must first become familiar with him. In this instance, that means gaining a thorough understanding of the factors that are affecting your performance. Once you've achieved that understanding, you'll, in turn, have greater appreciation for the way we've designed the training and nutritional portions of this book. So without further ado, let's take a closer look at the four major obstacles your genetics pose to you in the weight room. Remember, we presented them earlier; now it's time to expand upon them.

1. Fiber Type

There are several different types of human muscle fibers; some are better at producing strength and power, while others are better suited for endurance work. Care to take a stab as to

(continued on page 24)

ALTERNATIVE MEDICINE

In a perfect world, guys would be able to do all the exercises we recommend later in this book with no problem at all. Unfortunately, due to pre-existing injuries, equipment limitations, or just plain weakness, certain lifts might be out of the question, initially at least. We've therefore put together a preemptive list of acceptable alternatives you can use until you're able to include the real deal in your program.

EXERCISE »   **FRONT SQUAT & SQUAT**

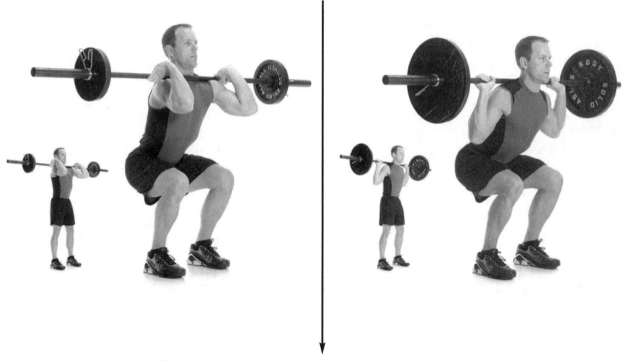

REPLACEMENT »   **LEG PRESS**

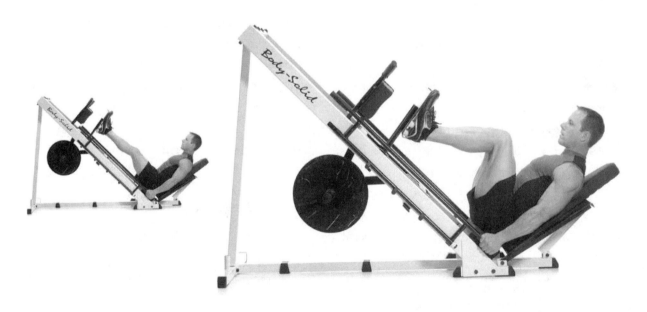

EXERCISE))   **DEADLIFT**

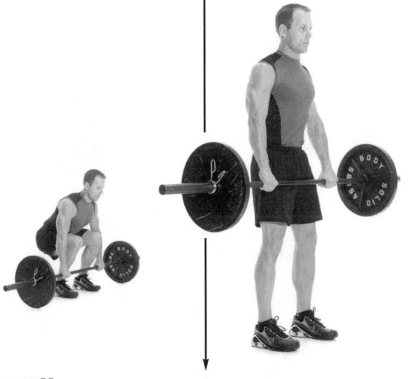

REPLACEMENT))   **LIMITED RANGE DEADLIFT**
(done off supports in a
squat rack, or off blocks)

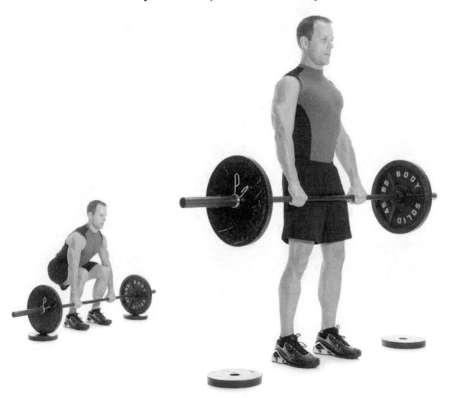

(continued)

EXERCISE ❯❯　　　　　　　　　**PULLUP**

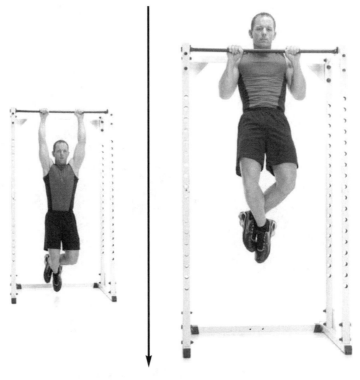

REPLACEMENT ❯❯　　　　**NEGATIVE PULLUP**
(use a stool or chair to boost yourself
up over the bar and lower yourself
for 5 to 8 seconds per repetition)

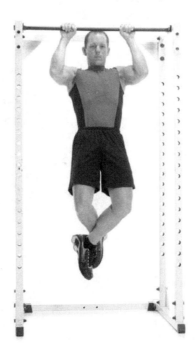

DIPS

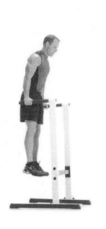

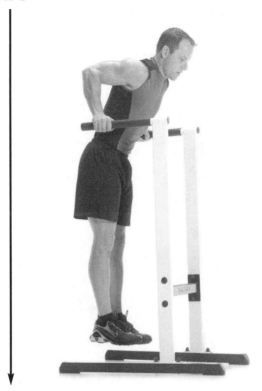

CROSS BENCH DIPS

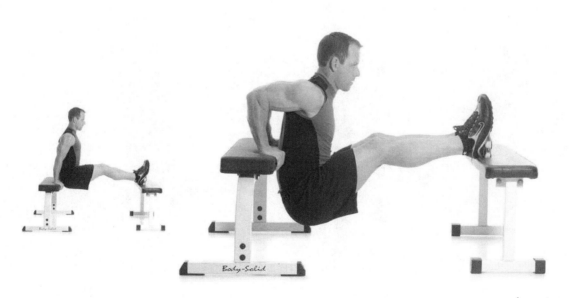

(continued)

EXERCISE »   **CLEAN & PRESS**

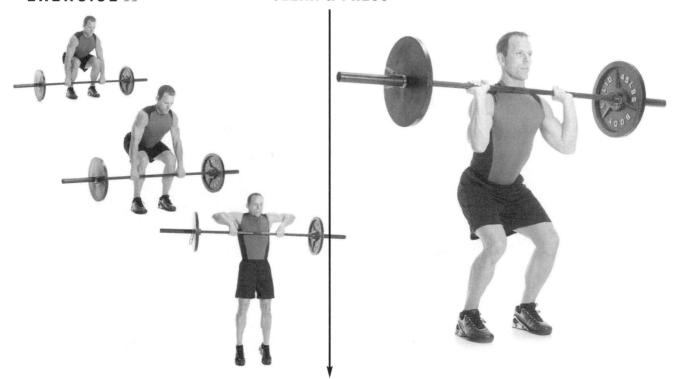

REPLACEMENT »

**HAMMER CURL
TO AN OVERHEAD PRESS**

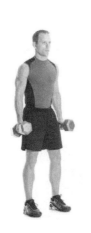

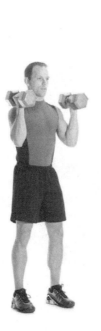

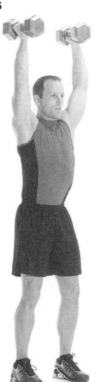

EXERCISE)) GLUTE HAM RAISE

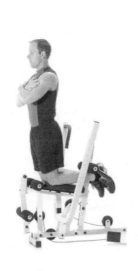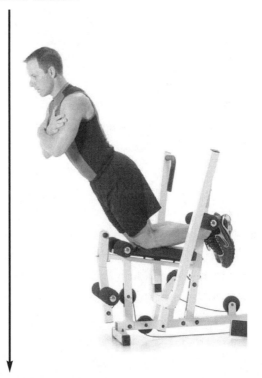

REPLACEMENT)) UNILATERAL BACK EXTENSION

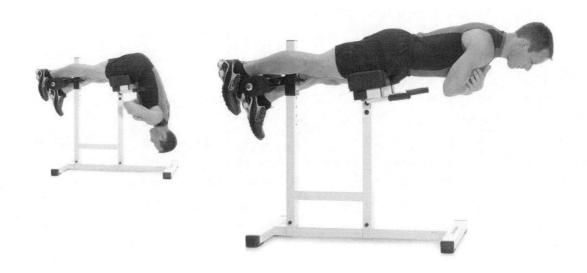

DIFFERENT STROKES FOR SKINNY FOLKS

which is likely predominant in ectomorphs? If you picked the kind that is great for endurance (fatigue resistant) yet poor at generating strength and power (force), give yourself a star. Slow-twitch muscle fibers are the endurance kind, and boy, do they live up to their name. Their healthy supply of blood and oxygen allows them to recover quickly, making them perfect for endurance activities such as walking, jogging, and maintaining posture (something some muscles have gotta do all day long). Unfortunately, they contract about as quickly as your grandfather getting out of an easy chair, placing you at a distinct disadvantage when it comes to strength and power activities such as jumping, sprinting, and weight training.

We'll get into fiber types and the impact they have on your ability to build muscle in much greater detail in Chapter 4 when we discuss training frequency. For now though, realize that having a larger proportion of slow-twitch fibers isn't exactly ideal when it comes to increasing size and strength. Besides generating little force and being so slow to contract, they also have the least potential for hypertrophy (muscle growth) of the three major fiber types. Sure, they're great for endurance activities, but their superior ability to utilize oxygen is of little help when you're pinned at the bottom of the bench press!

However, it's not as hopeless as it may seem. Even if you do possess a higher-than-average proportion of slow-twitch fibers, you can still build significant amounts of muscle mass. After all, no one has only slow-twitch fibers. Even the best world-class endurance athletes still have 40 percent fast-twitch fibers, and these fibers are the ones that can be targeted for growth. The program presented in this book does just that—target those fast-twitch fibers for hypertrophy.

2. Limb Length

Want to hear something that will make ectomorphs everywhere shudder? Long limbs and heavy weights are a bad combination. Long limbs force you to move the load you're handling through a much larger range of motion than someone with shorter limbs. Remember that the next time your stubby-armed buddy starts chirping about how much he can bench. His short limbs have to travel through only a short range of motion, making bench presses much easier.

Besides making you work harder, your long limbs can also place some extra strain on your joints and connective tissue by altering the mechanics of your new staple lifts such as the squat, bench press, and deadlift. Yet we're about to suggest doing all three lifts anyway. You see, in Chapter 3, we're going to teach you some tricks for altering your technique just enough to make these otherwise difficult lifts more "ectomorph friendly." We'll break these lifts down in painstaking detail, showing you specific ways to make them both safer and more effective. Simple changes such as improving flexibility and altering the width of your grip or stance can make a dramatic difference in the amount of weight you can handle and the safety of that load.

3. Metabolism

Ectomorphs are famous for their remarkably speedy metabolisms. If you've ever heard someone say that their metabolism is so fast that they can eat whatever they want without gaining weight, you can bet they're either an exercise addict or an ectomorph.

But while it's common to think that the ectomorph has a screaming baseline resting metabolic rate, unless there's an underlying thyroid hyperactivity, ectomorphs probably don't have remarkably different resting metabolisms than the rest of us. So what gives? Well, the answer's pretty NEAT—literally. NEAT stands for nonexercise activity thermogenesis, and it could explain why ectos have such a difficult time gaining weight. We all know that vigorous exercise burns a lot of calories, but apparently there's a lot to be said for the amount of calories you burn during everyday tasks such as running errands, doing laundry, and even fidgeting. According to a recent study, it seems that some people are better at this than others. Researchers fed a group of 16 normal adults an additional 1,000 calories above their daily energy needs. Although the average weight gain for the group was 10 pounds, the amount of weight gained per individual varied from 2, all the way up to almost 16 pounds!

Interestingly, because all of the subjects were similar in terms of both basal metabolic rate (metabolism while lying in bed and not moving) and the energy burned during the digestive processes, the differences in weight gain were attributed to varying rates of NEAT. In fact, it's been estimated that subjects less likely to gain weight when overfeeding can burn up to 69 percent of the excess energy intake as heat. That means there's not much left for storage as fat.

Of course, an elevated metabolism, regardless of its explanation, is only part of the equation. It's been our experience that most ectomorphs simply undereat when trying to gain size. We consult with ectos all the time who tell us that they "eat like a horse," or "eat everything in sight" only to recall a diet that barely has enough calories to sustain a gerbil, a really *small* gerbil. What they fail to realize is that it's not just about how often or how much they need to eat; it's also about the quality of the nutrients they're taking in. Who cares if you eat six times a day if your diet consists mainly of snack foods and anything off the dollar menu at Mickey

D's? Both the amount and the diversity of food you'll be eating on our program are going to be a far cry from what you're putting into your body now. Trust us though; the results will be worth it in the end.

4. Muscle/Tendon Length Relationships

Another crucial factor in determining your ultimate potential to build size and strength is the length of your muscles in relation to your tendons (tendons hold muscles and bones together). Generally speaking, longer muscles are stronger than shorter muscles because they have a greater cross-sectional area (i.e., they've got more protein capable of generating force).

But stop! We know what you're thinking. You're long and lean, so your muscles must be long too, right? Nice try. Ectomorphs are actually known for shorter muscles with notoriously long tendons. So just because your limbs are long, that doesn't mean your muscles are, too. So what's wrong with short muscles? Well, besides the reduced cross-sectional area inherent to short muscles, you've got those long tendons, which don't quite bulk up either.

One advantage the long-tendoned have, though, lies in the fact that the placement of those tendons, i.e., where they attach to bone, can help enhance strength development. Although tendons just don't have the growth potential of muscles, if those tendons are long and insert far away from the axis of rotation around a joint, they'll contribute greatly to strength. Need an example? Here's one. Let's say you have two guys doing a barbell biceps curl. The first guy has a biceps tendon that inserts 1 inch from his elbow. The second guy, though, has a tendon that inserts 1.5 inches from his elbow. That little bit of a difference is enough to give the second

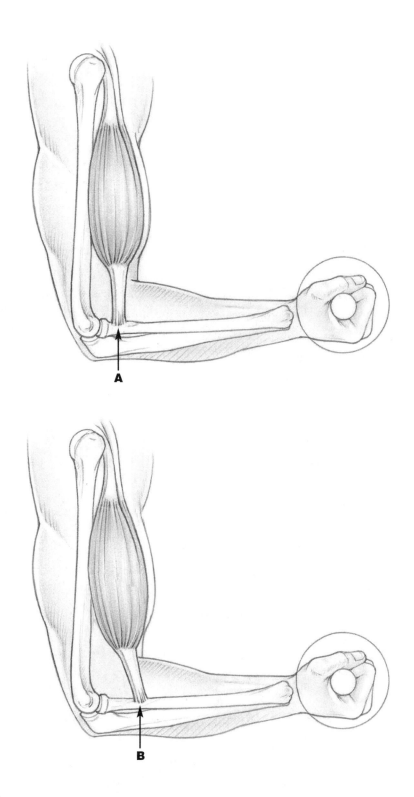

The lifter on the top (tendon in position A) would have a biomechanical advantage over the lifter on the bottom (tendon in position B) due to the tendon inserting a little farther away from the joint.

guy a significant biomechanical advantage to lift that weight. So those long tendons, while potentially impairing overall mass development, can be a big help in your quest to get stronger.

THE ROAD LESS TRAVELED

Just because you have to march to the beat of a different drummer and garner your information from alternative sources doesn't mean that you're in any way inferior to those who succeed with the more mainstream approach. It just means that you have to take a different path. We'll be the first to admit that it's quite a change to train in such a counterintuitive manner. But remember, most scrawny guys come to us desperate after trying "everything else" with limited success. So when we give them their new training and nutritional programs, while a bit skeptical at first, they're absolutely amazed at the progress they're able to achieve. They soon come to realize that breaking the shackles of skinnydom requires a completely different approach.

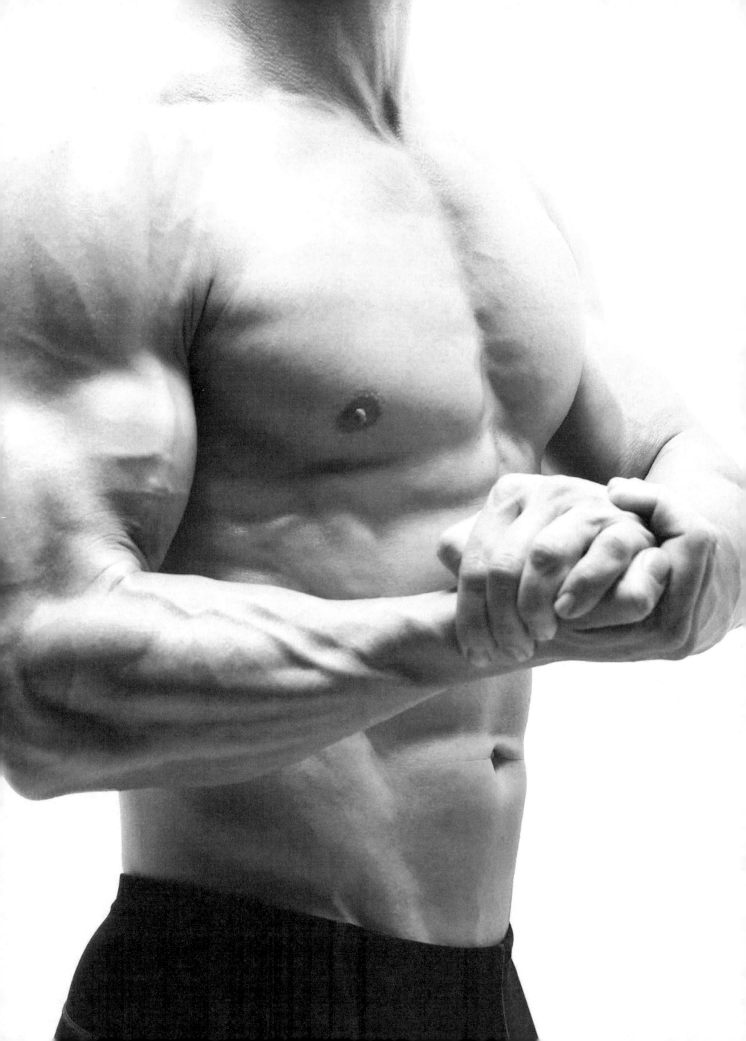

THREE THE *HARD* WAY

If you've been paying attention up until this point, you've probably noticed an interesting little paradox starting to develop. It seems that much of the advice aimed at guys in your situation centers around the importance of lifts such as the squat, deadlift, and bench press. Yet we just finished telling you that with your long limbs, these exercises, or at least two of them—the squat and the bench press—can be really difficult. So what's the deal?

The deal is that this perceived contradiction serves as one of our primary motives for writing this book. You see, although many authors suggest that ectomorphs simply get to the gym and increase their lifting loads in "the big three" exercises (squats, deadlifts, and bench press), they don't discuss the difficulties that ectomorphs undoubtedly face when trying to perform these with conventional form. Rather than make this mistake ourselves, we decided to devote this entire chapter to helping you learn how to most effectively execute these lifts to achieve maximum benefit.

Before we analyze these lifts in detail, we'd like to first address the double-edged sword they represent. On the plus side, because they require you to use such a large amount of muscle mass, the squat, deadlift, and bench press not only expose your body to heavier loading, but in doing so, promote the release of the all-natural muscle-building hormones such as growth hormone and testosterone into your bloodstream. Try as you might, it's difficult to create a similar effect with biceps curls and lateral raises, primal screams that often accompany these lifts notwithstanding. On the down side, however, those same heavy loads can also put a tremendous amount of strain on joints and connective tissue, a strain that is only amplified by improper technique. But wait, here's the real kicker. Depending on your degree of "ectomorphy" (as measured in Chapter 1), your basic body structure may in fact lend itself to increased strain rates, despite your diligence to execute these lifts with proper form!

Take the bench press, for instance. This lift looks simple enough. Lie down on bench, grasp bar, lower across chest, and press back up. A closer look, however, reveals that there's much more to it than that. This holds especially true when performing the bodybuilding-style bench press favored in most gyms. Using a standard shoulder-width grip and lowering the bar across the midline of the chest places quite a strain on the shoulder joint, a problem only made worse by having long arms. Similar difficulties also exist with the traditional barbell squat. Long femurs (upper thigh bones) combined with a short torso can cause you to lean forward excessively, placing increased strain on the lower back. Add in what is typically insufficient flexibility in the lower body, and you have all the makings of a visit to the chiropractor.

So what's the answer? Ditch these most hallowed of lifts, and try your luck at putting on some size with machines and isolation exercises? Or take the time to learn exactly where your weaknesses lie, and formulate strategies to combat them? Call us thickheaded, but we much prefer the second option. In this chapter, we'll show you just how to turn your sissy squat and puny press into strong, safe, and muscle-building lifts.

A PRESSING CONCERN

We figure the bench press is a pretty good place to start. After all, trying to find a guy who doesn't want to increase his bench is like trying to find a guy who doesn't want a date with Britney Spears. Unfortunately, though, since Britney hasn't been returning your calls, chances are you're going to have to settle for pressing a few more pounds.

The interesting thing about the bench press is that there are so many different ways to do it. Depending on the angle you use (incline, flat, or decline), your grip width (close, medium, or wide), and where you keep your elbows in relation to your torso, you can alter the lift dramatically. The key, however, is finding a variation that's best suited to

you biomechanically, rather than allowing popular opinion to dictate the way you execute the lift.

To better understand what we mean, a little anatomy lesson is order. The chest, or pectoralis major, actually has two heads, a sternocostal head, which originates at the costal cartilage on top of the first six ribs and the adjoining portion of the sternum, and a clavicular head, which originates at the middle portion of the clavicle (collarbone). Both heads then fuse together into a common tendon that inserts on the humerus (upper arm bone). We mention this because much is often made about the impact that factors such as bench angle and grip width have on different parts of the pecs. Some say that the incline bench press hits the upper pecs, while decline hits the lower pecs. Interestingly, scientific studies of both the clavicular and sternocostal heads during incline, flat, and decline presses have yielded mixed results. Some studies have found no significant difference in upper pec activation between the different pressing angles, while others show that close grip incline and wide grip flat presses do indeed increase upper and lower pec activation, respectively. In the end, the differences between movements, in terms of chest activation, are small. The difference in pectoral activation you'll get from various forms of benching pales in comparison to the benefit you'll receive from simply focusing on lifting the most weight you can in the most biomechanically efficient manner possible. The point here is that you needn't be overly concerned with "blasting your pecs from a variety of angles." This idea is just something that the muscle mags like to toss around from time to time to keep things interesting.

So how does one alter the bench press to achieve optimal biomechanical efficiency? Well, for instance, as we mentioned previously, having long arms means that the bar has to travel through a greater range of motion. This essentially means that

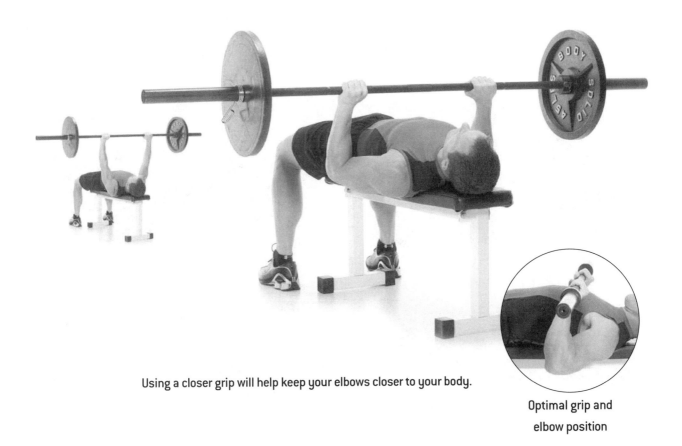

Using a closer grip will help keep your elbows closer to your body.

Optimal grip and
elbow position

you'll be doing much more work at a given weight than your stubby-armed friends. Naturally, this has led to the recommendation that in order for ectos to get the most out of the bench press, they should shorten the range of motion. While definitely a viable strategy, we feel that this is only part of the equation. After all, there are issues at the shoulder joint that need attention before loading up the bar and "benchin' heavy."

SHOULDERING THE LOAD

The version of the bench press you most often see involves the lifter using a grip that's slightly wider than shoulder's width and lowering the bar down across the midline of the chest. This is done in an effort to better target the pecs, because it takes much of the onus off the front deltoids and triceps. Unfortunately, it also reduces the amount of space

between the head of the humerus (upper arm bone) and the acromion process (tip of the scapula). This junction is located at the shoulder joint. This position, especially if used repeatedly over time, can lead to shoulder impingement, a painful condition that's caused by tendons and ligaments being pinched between two bony structures. Simply put, it's an extremely biomechanically inefficient position to lift from. So naturally, the obvious question is "if it's so bad for you, why does everyone bench that way?" One word: tradition.

For as long as either of us can remember, the benching technique described above has been the one most often featured in books, magazine articles, and of course, weight rooms far and wide. Chances are, you've been benching this way ever since you got your first weight set back in high school. A pity, really, especially considering how

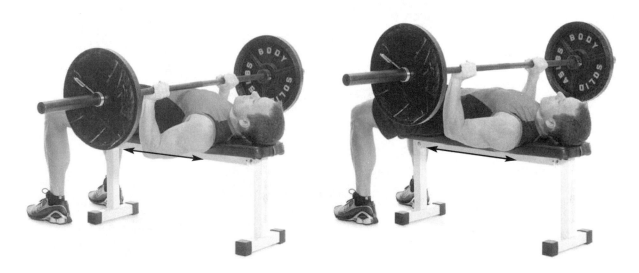

Going too low *(left)* puts unnecessary strain on the shoulder joint. Keep your elbows in line with your torso *(right)*.

much time and effort you could have saved yourself by benching in a manner more conducive to your physique. While using a wide grip position with the elbows flared away from your body may reduce shoulder and tricep involvement, it doesn't exactly put the chest in an optimal position to develop force. Add in the fact that your shorter muscle bellies and longer tendons need to stretch farther to reach their point of attachment on the humerus (upper arm bone), and it's no wonder that most ectomorphs have got the bench press of a prepubescent girl.

So how should the ectomorph perform the bench press? Well, one way to combat the problems mentioned above is to simply use a slightly narrower grip. Now, we're not talking about doing a close grip bench press here. Rather, we're talking about moving your grip in just enough so that the elbows are closer to your trunk. While it's true that a closer grip will increase the contribu-

tion of your triceps and front deltoids, it also gives the chest a better angle of pull. Don't believe us? Try this little test.

Hold your right arm straight out to your side, parallel to the floor. Next, place your left hand on your right pec, and try to contract your chest. Not much going on, eh? Try it again, but this time lower your arm to about 45 degrees (so your fingers are pointed diagonally toward the floor). Feel the difference? Now do you suppose perhaps that you might be able to handle a little more weight if you benched with your elbows in closer to your body? Plus, you'll get the added benefit of knowing you're not tearing your shoulders apart.

While this elbow thing is a huge help, it's not all you've got to be concerned with. After all, keeping your elbows in closer to your body doesn't change the length of your arms. That's right; we've still got the whole range-of-motion issue to deal with. Besides the length of the humerus, two other factors

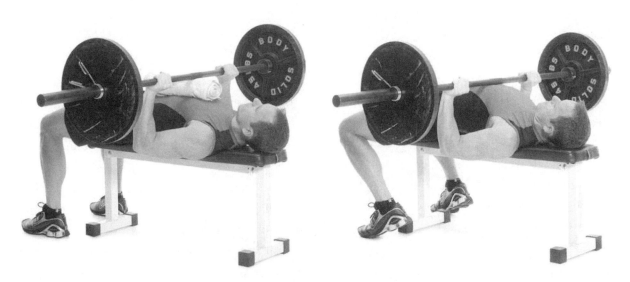

Two techniques for shortening the range of motion include placing a towel on the chest *(left)* or arching your back and lifting your rib cage up higher *(right)*.

ectomorphs have working against them on the bench press are rib-cage size and forearm length. We know, it sounds a little weird, but bear with us. Typically, lifters who excel at the bench press have big barrel chests and relatively short arms. The advantage this gives them is that because their rib cage sits up higher off the bench, they don't have to lower the weight as far. Combined with their relatively short forearms, this helps keep strain off the shoulder joint by forcing the pecs to do more of the work. Here's why.

In the bottom position of the bench press, the depth of your elbows in relation to your torso has a lot to do with where the majority of the stress is being applied. When you have a large rib cage that sits up high off the bench and short forearms, at the bottom of the range, your elbows will be either even with, or only *slightly* past the level of the bench. In this position, you're effectively reducing the amount of stretch being placed

on the shoulder-joint capsule and in turn keeping most of the stress on your pecs. Conversely, having a shallower rib cage and long forearms will require you to lower the bar much farther to reach the same point, thus causing the elbows to dip down well beneath your torso. This is simply not a good idea for most people because once the shoulder-joint capsule has been stretched, it loses its ability to stabilize the shoulder under a load, setting you up for a whole slew of injuries.

Therefore, if increasing the workload on the pecs (and maintaining a healthy shoulder joint) is the goal, it makes sense to shorten the range of motion. But don't go hacking off your lower forearm just yet. Rather, you can achieve this same goal by placing a couple of small boards or a rolled-up bath towel across your chest. You then simply use this as a reference point for how far to lower the bar. Another effective strategy and one that is favored by power-lifters is to pinch your shoulder blades together tightly, and bring the bar slightly below the nipple line (to the xyphoid process) at the base of the sternum. Retracting your shoulder blades in this manner, kind of like you'd do when performing a seated row, requires you to actively contract the muscles of the upper back, thus adding support and stability to the posterior aspect (rear) of the shoulder girdle.

This not only gives you a stronger platform to drive the weight from, but when combined with driving your feet into the floor and slightly arching your back, it allows you to effectively shorten the range that the weight must travel through. Decreasing the space between your shoulder blades and your hips raises your torso slightly, thus not requiring you to lower the bar as far. Plus, it allows you to keep most of the onus on the pecs, front deltoids, and triceps where it belongs.

Now, before you get on us about excessively arching the back, keep in mind that if the hips always remain in contact with the bench, this prevents excessive arching. The pelvic thrust is not part of the bench press, and if you save your thrusting for non-gym-related activities, your back should be fine. We should, however, mention that those of you with a history of lower back problems should probably take a pass on this latter technique, and stick with placing something on your chest (such as the rolled-up towel discussed earlier) to shorten the range of motion.

Although limiting your range of motion and keeping your elbows in closer to your body will result in heavier loads and decreased shoulder strain, it's not as if the barbell bench press is all you need to build up your chest. Things such as dips, dumbbell presses (because they allow you to alter the range of motion), and even flys all have their place. Remember, it's not that ectomorphs *can't* or shouldn't do isolation exercises. Rather, the ectomorph should not make these types of exercise the focal point of their program. Performed with the proper modifica-

tions, the barbell bench press is an extremely effective lift. Just be aware that despite its lofty status in the exercise hierarchy, it's not the only game in town when it comes to building up your chest.

YOU DON'T KNOW SQUAT

The squat has been called the "king of all exercises." It's a lift that is virtually unparalleled in terms of its ability to bring about improvements in strength and power. Unfortunately, to some, it also carries with it the stigma of being "dangerous." Some say that it places unnecessary strain on the knees and lower back. But the truth is, it only does so if you're using more weight than you can handle, and/or sloppy form. The fact is, when done properly, the squat is among the safest and most effective exercises you can do. Anyone who tells you otherwise needs to get his facts straight. Perhaps you could recommend that they read this book or visit us at www.scrawnytobrawny.com.

That said, just as with the bench press, the squat is an exercise that needs some tweaking to be most effective for you ectomorphs. Much the same way the length of your arms presented a problem with the bench press, those stilt-like legs of yours can make squatting a real adventure. And, if those long legs just happen to be accompanied by a short torso, it makes things all the more interesting. Not only do you have to move the weight through a larger range of motion, but the length of your legs in relation to your torso can cause you to lean forward at the waist much farther than someone with shorter limbs. But before you dismiss your inability to squat effectively as some biomechanical inevitability, let's take a closer look at what's going on, starting from the ground up.

Take a Stand

It's just like the old adage says, you can't build on a weak foundation. Well, you can; it's just that

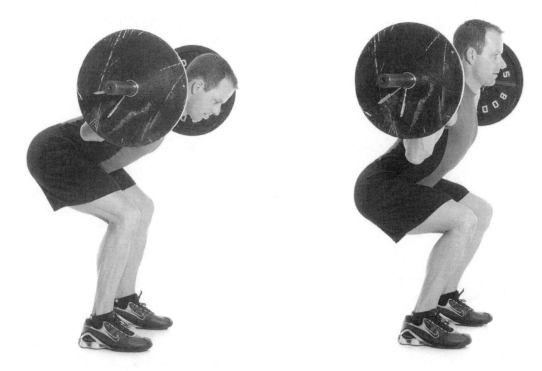

Keep a wide stance and reduce your forward lean while squatting.
The photo on the left shows an incorrect stance and the photo on the right shows the proper form.

you probably won't be too thrilled with the results. In terms of the squat, when you think foundation, think stance. Because, believe it or not, the type of stance you take is going to have a major impact on the way you perform the lift. Typically, most lifters opt for a stance that's slightly wider than shoulder's width apart, although there are those who feel more comfortable with either a narrower or wider foot placement. The stance is important because it determines your range of motion and where the stress of the movement will fall. More on this in a moment.

Another important factor to consider is the direction that your feet are pointing. Along with stance width, foot placement helps determine the range of motion around the hip joint and, in turn, affects the type of load you can handle. Again, foot placement and stance width also determine which

segments of the lower body are stressed to a greater degree.

Now, don't make the mistake of thinking that we're discussing the vague and unproven bodybuilding folklore that tells us that turning the feet in different directions will activate different areas within the four main quadriceps (thigh) muscles. Rather, we want to impress upon you the idea that the right combination of stance and foot position will help you stay more upright, thus keeping the majority of the stress on the quads, hamstrings, and glutes, and off the spinal erectors (lower back). It would be different if you were a powerlifter with the objective of moving as much weight as possible. In that case, sticking that ol' rump out would be just fine, since it recruits those hips and spinal erectors like nobody's business. However, seeing as how there aren't a whole lot of ectomorphic powerlifters, and considering that your primary reason for even attempting to squat is likely to build up your thighs without hurting yourself in the process, the more upright you can remain, the better off you're going to be.

The first way to improve your upright posture in the squat is to use a wider stance (when we say wider, we typically mean a stance in which your feet are placed approximately 4 to 6 inches outside your shoulders). The reason that a wider stance allows you to remain more upright is that it essentially shortens the distance the bar and your body must travel by reducing the amount of hip displacement relative to your feet and the weight. Think of it this way: If you were to stand to the side of someone and analyze the "parallel" position of their squat (don't worry, we'll address the whole depth issue shortly), you should be able to draw a straight line from the center of the barbell, right through the center of the foot. During a normal squat, in relation to this line, the hips and butt will be shifted back behind the bar and foot position to a pretty significant degree. Now, if you're an ectomorph and have long upper legs, the popular narrow/shoulder width stance will require an even greater displacement of the hips and butt. It should come as no surprise that as the hips and butt shift back, the more forward lean you're going to have. With a big load on your back and a big forward lean, you're going to be subjected to what's called a "shearing force" in the lower back. Sections of the lumbar spine (L4 and L5, to be exact) located right around the waist level will be particularly prone to this stress if you've got a big forward lean going on. So, to reduce your forward lean, squat with a bit wider stance.

As for what role the position of the feet play in all of this, adopting a slight toe out position (where the left foot would be pointing to 11 o'clock and the right at 1 o'clock on an imaginary clock)

changes the position of the head of the femur (thigh bone) in the hip socket. This position allows for greater range of motion and will often feel more comfortable to those with longer femurs. Ectomorphs love this little trick because it allows them to squat down lower without the hips feeling so restricted. It should be mentioned, however, that this increased freedom of movement should in no way act as a substitute for increasing flexibility in those muscles around the hips that may be tight, most specifically in this instance, the hip flexors and TFL (tensor fascia latae). Tightness in these muscles can lead to a restricted range of motion in the squat exercise and an excessive forward lean (we'll show you how to stretch these little buggers in Chapter 6). We've had tremendous success in helping ectomorphs improve their range of motion through flexibility enhancement. Add this newfound flexibility and an altered stance (a bit wider than normal) and foot position (slightly turned out), and the squat becomes magically transformed into a more ectomorph-friendly exercise.

Since we're on the topic of flexibility, perhaps now would be a good time to address another major concern of you long-legged lifters. Namely, the flexibility (or lack thereof) around the ankle joint. It's been argued by some that people with long femurs in relation to their torso quickly begin to exhaust range of motion at the ankle as they descend into a squat, especially during a typical high-bar bodybuilding-style squat. This means that as they squat down, their ankle flexibility begins to become the limiting factor for the depth of their squat. When this happens, the only way to get lower is to lean farther forward, something we've been cautioning you against. Once the forward lean is pronounced enough, the heels have to come off the ground, and this is a major no-no. If you find yourself excessively leaning forward when you squat, or you find your heels coming up off the ground consistently, you might need to perform some flexibility work at the hips and certainly at the ankle. Most ectomorphs do. How much flexibility work depends on how you squat and how long your femurs are.

If your femurs are only slightly longer than your torso, and you're diligent about stretching to increase the range of motion in both your ankles and hips, so long as you don't squat much deeper than parallel, you should be fine. On the other hand, if your physique has more of that "man on stilts" look to it, regardless of how good you are about stretching, you'll likely need to cut your squats somewhat short of this position when performing the traditional back squat. Of course, you could always place a couple of weight plates, or a wooden block underneath your heels, but this really just serves as a crutch for inadequate flexibility. Besides, as you'll soon read, there are other options at your disposal.

A *Kneed* to Know Basics

As we start to pan our way up the body from the ankles, the next area we need to focus on when discussing the squat is the knee. The two main things we're going to concern ourselves with here are how far the knees should come forward in relation to the toes, and how they should be aligned in relation to the hips and feet. Each of these variables can have a tremendous impact on both the safety and effectiveness of the lift. As far as the forward movement of the knee goes, the farther the knee extends past the toes, the greater the shearing force the knee will be subjected to. Shearing force is simply a fancy term for the force that connective tissues (tendons and ligaments) experience when two bony structures slide across each other. In a healthy knee, as long as the person doesn't bounce or jerk to get out of the bottom position and can also keep his heels on the floor throughout the lift, this force on the

knee shouldn't pose much of a problem. If however, you have any sort of pre-existing knee pain or diagnosed knee condition, whether chronic or acute, allowing the knees to shoot past the toes might cause pain or even injury. Simply put, if squatting to a certain depth hurts, stop doing it, and consult a sports medicine expert immediately.

The other thing to watch for is how the knees "track," or stay in line with the direction of the hips and feet throughout the lift. Knees that pinch in or bow out during a squat need some help. Either there are muscle groups that are too tight and are pulling the knee out of alignment, or there are underlying muscle weaknesses that need to be addressed, or both. Whatever the case, a knee that fails to follow in the same direction as the foot is pointed is placing some major strain on joints and connective tissue. More often than not, the fix for this is as simple as some targeted flexibility work and unilateral (training one side at a time) strengthening to eliminate any underlying muscular weaknesses/imbalances that may exist. The self-assessment in Chapter 6 will help you identify and subsequently correct any flaws in your squatting technique.

In continuing our ascent of the body, the next stop is the upper torso and the issue of bar placement. Keep in mind, if you think we've skipped anything from a form perspective, hold your horses. The idea of this chapter is to point out some common errors and help you execute the squat more effectively. You'll find that step-by-step breakdown you're looking for later in the book. For now, let's discuss where you should place the bar and why. For bar placement, there are two options. The first option is known as the high bar, or bodybuilding-style squat. With this variation, the bar is placed up high across the trapezius. The high-bar squat forces a lifter to remain more upright in the torso, so as to better target the quads. Then, of course there's always the low bar, or powerlifting-style

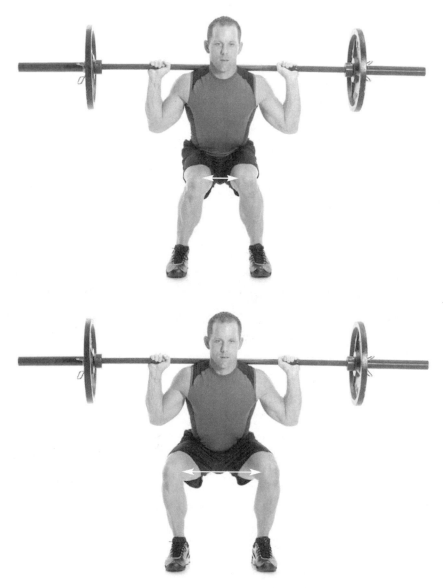

Squatting with knees pinching in or out is a recipe for disaster. These are both incorrect stances.

squat in which the bar sits lower down the upper back, on or near the tops of the shoulder blades. With this variation, the glutes, hamstrings, and spinal erectors are forced to work much harder due to the greater forward lean necessary to execute the lift.

Needless to say, if you're an ectomorph, neither one sounds all that appealing at first glance. After all, the low-bar style is *designed* to make you sit back, forcing you to lean way forward. And, with your long limbs and short torso, the high-bar vari-

ation has the potential to do the same. Sound hopeless? Well, it's not.

There are actually several things you can do to make the squat an effective part of your training arsenal regardless of where you place the bar. The first, as we've already mentioned, is to be diligent about improving your flexibility. You'd be surprised at how different the lift can feel by simply improving the range of motion of the muscles that surround the hips, knees, and ankles. Another thing that can help quite a bit is limiting your depth.

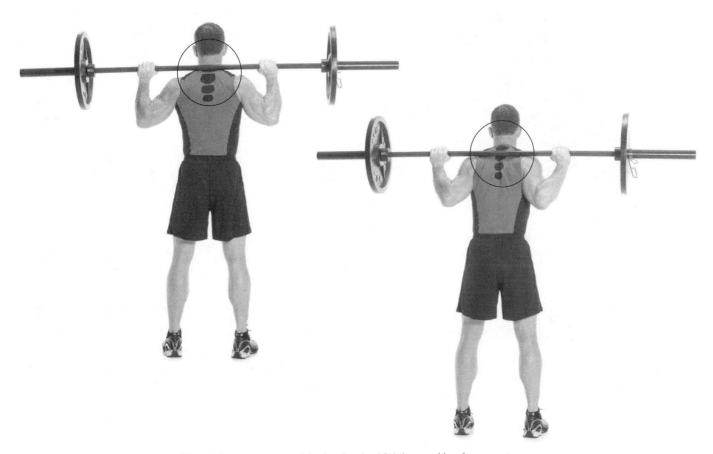

These show correct positioning for the high bar and low bar squat.

Now mind you, we're both huge proponents of the deep squat—in some situations. As long as a lifter possesses the balanced strength and flexibility to execute this movement properly, doesn't bounce to propel himself out of the bottom position, and has no pre-existing knee or lower back injuries, deep squats are about as effective a muscle-building exercise as there is. As good as they are, though, they don't make a whole lot of sense for taller lifters. Even if you are able to improve your range of motion and remain more upright, at some point, your basic body structure is going to require you to deviate from proper form. Once you do, the risk of injury to the knees and lower back increases dramatically. Besides which, once you pass parallel, the contribution of the glutes becomes that much greater. Seeing as how glute activation is the least of

your problems, and the objective is to get your quads working harder, limiting the range only makes sense from both a safety and practicality standpoint.

So how low should you go? We prefer to see the torso not exceed a 45-degree angle to the floor. Any more than that, and the lower back ends up bearing the brunt of the load. The trick is learning exactly how far down you can go without surpassing this 45-degree position. This may require the use of a friend or training partner to observe or possibly even videotape you as you execute the squat. Once you learn where to stop, it won't be long before you can perform the lift on your own. However, bear in mind that as you continue to work on improving your flexibility, you may, in fact, increase your depth slightly without increasing

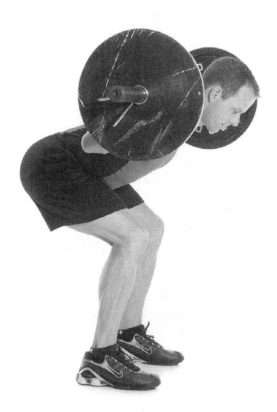

This is a squat with an excessive forward lean.

the degree of forward lean. This is highly individualized, though, and will probably only lead to minimal improvements in those with really long femurs.

Finally, it should be mentioned that when it comes to leg development, the traditional barbell squat isn't your only option. And no, in case you're wondering, this isn't where we try to make a case for the Smith machine. In our view, doing an exercise on the Smith machine is a poor substitute for doing its free-weight complement. True, in the case of the squat, it does allow you to maintain a more upright posture when squatting, regardless of your limb length. It does so, however, by forcing your body to adapt to the linear path in which the bar travels. Trouble is, that's not the way your body moves. By following this preset bar path, you end up placing too much stress on certain joints. The joint that takes on the brunt of this stress is the

knee. The poor thing is subjected to increased shearing forces as a result of suboptimal hamstring activation during the Smith machine squat.

Now that leaves the leg press, right? Well, the leg press *is* better. But not much. Sure, it allows you to handle more weight in a nice, back-supported position without placing the same shearing forces on the knee that the Smith machine does. But be careful of your lower back on this movement. Those of you who've ever gone down just a bit too low with a heavy load know exactly what we mean.

So by now, you must be thinking that we've eliminated all the good exercises. Without Smith machine squats and leg presses, what does that leave? Well, you're forgetting one of the absolute best exercises for quadriceps (thigh) development, the front squat. Aw, stop your whining. We know they're tough. We also know that because of where you support the bar, they require you to remain far more upright than the traditional barbell back squat. This is the huge benefit; no excessive forward lean here.

Now, many trainees we've spoken with complain that they can't do front squats properly, and that's why they avoid them. Yes, they are tough on an inflexible wrist. And yes, done improperly, the bar can cause some discomfort in those delicate shoulders. But don't worry, later in the book, we'll demonstrate a method of doing them that should solve all of your problems.

In addition to the front squat, there's always the box squats. With these, we once again borrow a page from our powerlifting friends. Although they do require you to sit back a bit more than regular squats, because you're actually sitting back on a box, the controlled motion will prevent some of the shearing stresses associated with a standard squat. Also, if your box is tall enough, you'll find the load on the spinal erectors is more manageable. However, since we want to focus on the quads here, and

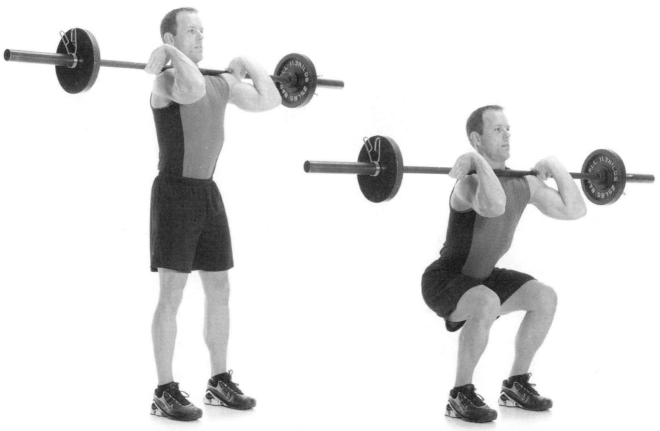

This is a proper front squat.

box squats use more glutes and hamstrings, we've gotta balance this exercise with the front squats described above as well as one-legged squats, split squats, and even Bulgarian split squats, if you're feeling really ambitious. All of these movements are compound, and all guaranteed to absolutely blast your legs. So, from this point forward, there's no more making excuses for why your legs won't grow. Work on improving your flexibility, strengthen any existing imbalances, and as long as the nutritional support is there, those twigs will turn into tree trunks in no time.

A DEADLIFT?

Ever wonder why you don't see many people doing deadlifts? Two reasons:

1. Deadlifts are brutally hard. It's tough to imagine another lift besides the squat that's as physically draining as the dead-lift. And, as we've already established, the more difficult the lift, the less inclined people are to do it.

2. Unfortunately, like the squat, the deadlift also has a reputation for being somewhat perilous.

Now, don't get us wrong; if you suffer from a disk herniation or any other type of serious lower back ailment, attempting to pick a loaded barbell up off the floor probably isn't a good idea, regardless of what your form looks like. Orthopedic limitations notwithstanding, however, the deadlift is pretty tough to beat when it comes to building strength and mass.

As if that last statement in and of itself isn't enough motivation to get your skinny butt deadlifting, try this on for size. The deadlift may actually be the one "big three" lift where those long limbs of

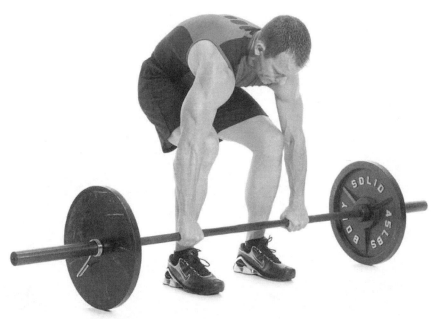

Deadlifting disaster: lifting with a rounded back

yours serve as a help rather than a hindrance. But before you get too giddy, you have to realize that this depends largely on the type of deadlift you do and what kind of form you use while doing it.

Gonna Need Some *Back*-Up

Regardless of which type of deadlift you do, the prime movers involved in the deadlift are the muscles of the posterior chain, namely the glutes, hamstrings, and spinal erectors (lower back). However, depending on which variation you opt for, there can also be a tremendous amount of quad involve-

ment as well. Now, since the deadlift and the squat use many of the same muscles, some of you may be wondering why you should do both. Well, for starters, the way that the weight is positioned in relation to the body's center of gravity (i.e., in front of the body's center of gravity) causes a greater degree of forward lean in the torso when performing the deadlift. The forward lean isn't optimal for squatting because of the stress a forward lean causes the lower back when there's a bar on top of the spine. With the deadlift, though, a certain degree of forward lean is optimal.

SQUATTING, ECTOMORPH STYLE

>> Work on improving flexibility around the hips, knees, ankles, and lower back (see Chapter 6).

>> Be sure to correct any existing weaknesses/imbalances before you attempt any heavy loading.

>> To target the quads, use either a high-bar back squat, and do not surpass a 45-degree forward lean, or do front squats.

>> To target the glutes, hamstrings, and spinal erectors, try low-bar box squats.

>> Turning the toes out slightly can help improve range but shouldn't be used as a crutch for poor flexibility.

>> Regardless of the type of squat you do, opt for a stance width that is at least 4 to 6 inches outside your shoulders.

We say this because the deadlift involves a much greater upper body component than the squat. The fact that you have to hold the weight in your hands rather than support it across your trapezius requires an even greater utilization of your upper back musculature. In order to prevent your back from rounding due to the pull of the weight, you have to actively contract your upper back and work to maintain an arch in your lower back. This requires a strong contraction from all the back muscles (including the lats, rhomboids, trapezius rear deltoids, and spinal erectors). This means leg and back growth. But be careful not to let your ego get in the way. If the pull of the weight causes you to round your back during the lift, immediately lower the weight until you can maintain the proper position. Rounding the back excessively can shift the stress onto the spinal ligaments and separates the normal space between the vertebrae. This can increase the possibility of disk herniations, so don't round that back!

But hold on a minute here! Didn't we mention something about the deadlift being at least somewhat conducive to an ectomorphic body type? We did, with a caveat. We said that it depends on what style of deadlift you choose. Take the classic bent-leg deadlift, for example. The increased forward lean at the waist already increases hip and lower back involvement; throw in long femurs and a short torso, and well . . . you know what to expect. Think squatting is tough? Try attempting to pull a couple of hundred pounds off the floor without the benefit of any elastic recoil from having lowered the weight from above. Trust us; it's no day at the beach. The only saving grace is that your long arms actually end up making the lift somewhat easier by not requiring you to lean forward quite as much as someone with shorter limbs. Trouble is, because of where the weight is positioned, even though your long arms effectively shorten the range of motion

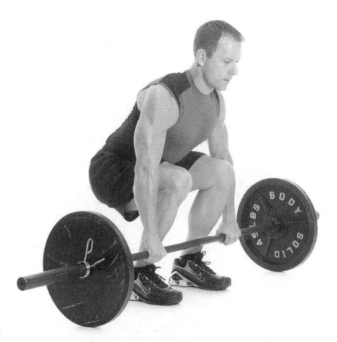

The right way to do a deadlift

somewhat, the advantage is once again minimized by those long femurs.

Typically what happens is that as you attempt to drive the weight off the floor using mainly your legs, the fact that your hips are displaced so far behind the bar makes it difficult to extend them optimally given the load. The quads, on the other hand, since they're easier for most people to recruit and are in a better position to develop force, end up extending the knee, which causes the hips to rise while still somewhat displaced behind the rest of the body. This "hip kick," as it's known, further increases shearing force on the lower back region. Instead, what you want is a simultaneous extension of the hips, knees, and spine as you lift the weight off the floor.

With the squat, inadequate flexibility created challenges for proper form. The same is true for the deadlift. Tight hamstrings, for instance, will cause the lower back to round (because it disallows the necessary lordoctic arch and forward tilt of the pelvis, for you anatomy buffs). Likewise, tight calf

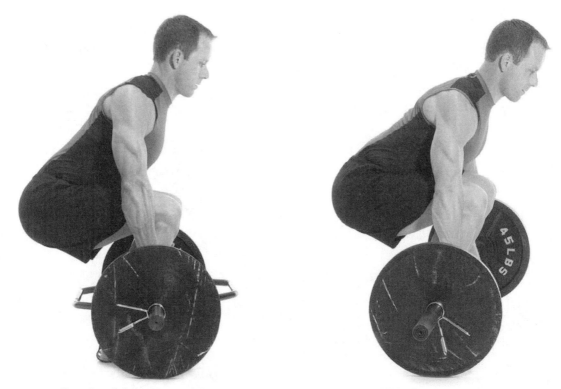

Note the slightly more upright posture used with the parallel grip deadlift pictured at left.

and hip musculature can exacerbate what is already a pretty pronounced forward lean, subjecting you to the risk of kicking up your hips. Obviously then, at the risk of starting to sound like a broken record, if you want to add deadlifts to your routine, or you want to improve your existing technique, flexibility work must be given an important priority.

In addition to performing flexibility work, the other thing that can dramatically improve your ability to execute the deadlift is to change the position of the weight in relation to your center of gravity. Enter the trap bar, a.k.a. parallel grip deadlift. This exercise can be done either with a specialized bar or dumbbells if you have enough flexibility. The major difference between the parallel grip and conventional deadlift is that with the former, because the weight is held next to your body as opposed to in front of it, it enables you to remain much more upright. This means much less forward lean and much greater quad activation. So much so, in fact, that the parallel grip deadlift is preferred by

some over the squat as their primary lower body lift. Those who are unable to execute the barbell squat due to either limited flexibility or previous injury often find that they can handle significant loads with the parallel grip deadlift. This is due to the fact that in addition to being able to remain more upright, their longer arms help shorten the range of motion.

Of course, it should be noted that as one works to improve flexibility, the range of parallel grip deadlifts can always be increased by performing the lift while standing on 25-pound weight plates, or a 4-inch wooden platform, or by using weights no larger than Olympic 25-pound plates to load the bar. Either way, you'll have to descend a bit farther to both initiate the lift-off phase and lower the weight back down to the floor. Using dumbbells is also another viable option, provided, of course, you have enough weight to challenge yourself throughout the lift. Regardless of which option you choose, the parallel grip deadlift is probably your best

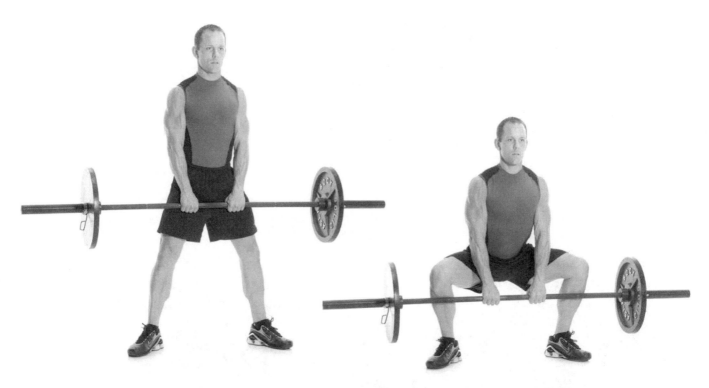

The sumo deadlift

option for safe and effective lower-body loading.

One last type of deadlift that warrants mention here is the sumo deadlift. Despite the fact that the bar is positioned in front of the body, the combination of a wide stance and significant amount of foot turnout allows you to remain much more upright. This results in greater lower-body activation and reduces the contribution of the lower back as compared with the conventional bent-leg deadlift. It should be noted, however, that in both variations, care must be taken to keep the bar as close to the body as possible. The more vertical the path of the bar, the less strain imposed on the lower back. Bear in mind, though, that for some of you, this may result in significant scraping of the shins and knees. Unfortunately, this is just something you'll have to get used to. Don't be one of those weenies who lets the bar travel out in front of your body to avoid contact with your legs. Personally, we'd choose roughed-up shins over disk surgery any day of the week. Besides, if it bothers you that much, just wear heavy sweats or thick tube/knee socks on deadlifting days.

At this point, you should now have a good working understanding of the biomechanical issues that you as an ectomorph must confront in attempting to include "the big three" in your program. Whether you choose to view these as either problems to be solved, or excuses to avoid, is really up to you. The simple fact is that these exercises and their derivatives are the ones that'll get you where you want to go. It's about time you stopped letting them kick your butt.

If you're confused about where each exercise and its variants should appear, don't sweat it. This chapter wasn't designed to teach you how to write a training program. That chapter comes later. Rather, this chapter is designed to give you the knowledge of the big three lifts that'll allow you to understand why they're placed where they are in the training program. They say that knowledge is power. Well if that's the case, you're now one powerful dude. Remember that the next time you feel that bar in your hands.

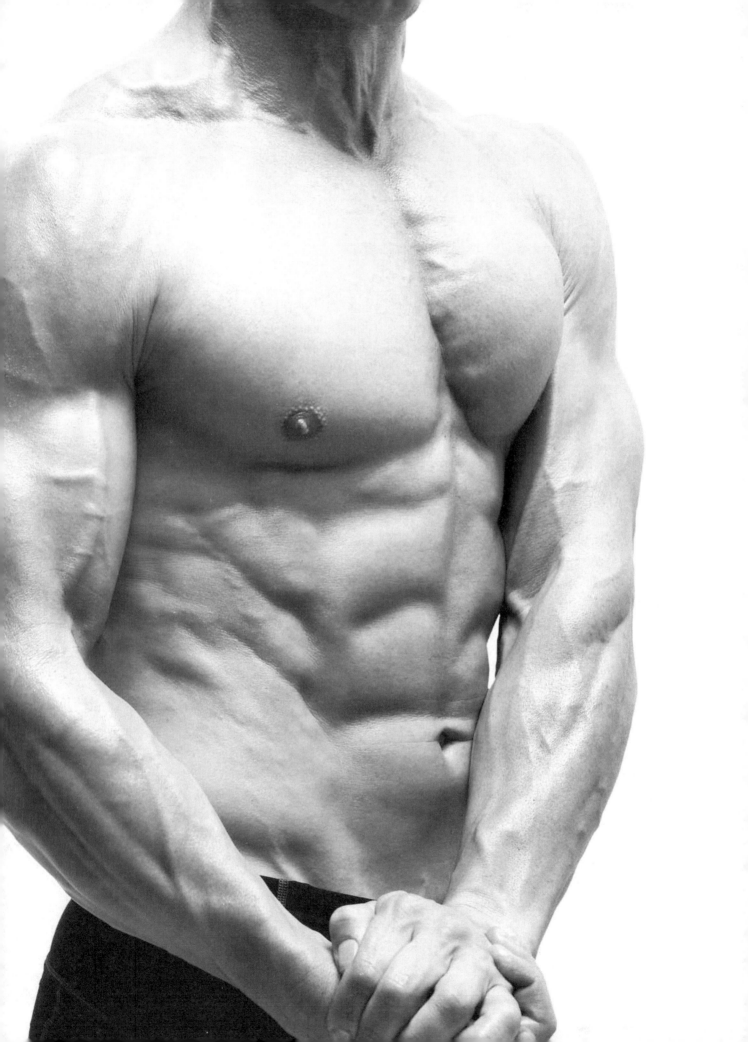

TRAINING:
HOW MUCH IS TOO MUCH?

》》While the previous chapter focused on "the big three" lifts, this chapter has got a big three of its own. These are "the big three" of muscle growth:

1. Train properly, with intensity.

2. Allow for adequate recovery time outside of the gym.

3. Provide the body with enough total energy and the right types of food.

Having one or two of "the big three" above is not enough. You need the whole trifecta to get bigger and stronger. However, seeing as how we've devoted half the book to nutrition, and get plenty detailed when it comes to training, we're going to focus mainly on the recovery aspect here. And by recovery, we mean the amount of rest you're taking between workouts.

While it's widely agreed that *adequate* recovery is essential for muscle growth, trying to assign a value to exactly what constitutes adequate can be a pretty daunting task. Besides all the of training and nutritional factors, you also have to consider things such as sleeping patterns, stress levels, and the amount of physical activity you engage in outside of the gym. Any one, or more likely a combination, of these factors can leave you on the wrong side of the recovery equation. Obviously, this is a bad place to be if you're looking to add more muscle to your frame.

Compounding this whole recovery conundrum is the fact that much of the advice currently available to guys in your situation is extremely generic. For instance, most hardgainer (there's that word again) training protocols call for brief, intense bouts of exercise with pretty long (read several days) recovery intervals between workouts. Many also advocate the minimization or, in some cases, outright elimination of cardiovascular exercise. In fact, it's not uncommon to see hardgainer routines that call for two

45-minute training sessions, or a whopping 90 minutes of intense physical activity per week! That's just slightly more exercise than the average couch potato gets and certainly not enough exercise to go from scrawny to brawny!

Not that we're implying that you should you start engaging in long, drawn-out training sessions every other day. In our experience, that approach seldom works for individuals who have a hard time building muscle. It's just that these recommendations seem rather broad to us and don't take into consideration things such as training phases, the number of calories you're consuming, and any supplementary physical activity you may be doing.

In our view, an ectomorph who has an office job, is consuming a sufficient number of calories, and is in the midst of a hypertrophy phase can afford to train more frequently than one who does manual labor all day and is engaged in a heavy strength phase. It's not about following some arbitrary guidelines; finding the proper training frequency is more a matter of understanding the factors that affect your body's recuperative powers.

DON'T GET TYPECAST

Back in Chapter 3, we pointed out a rather interesting paradox regarding those of you with more ectomorphic tendencies and your "need" versus your ability to perform lifts such as the squat, deadlift, and bench press. Well, it looks like we have another one to contend with, this time relating to muscle fiber types. Uh oh, we smell another physiology lesson coming. Don't worry, we promise to keep it brief.

You already know about the type I's (slow-twitch) and their impressive endurance capabilities. At the other end of the spectrum, you've got your type IIb fibers. Scientists call these fibers fast-twitch/glycolytic fibers because they contract quickly and use glucose (carbohydrates) as a primary source of energy. (Type I fibers are slow and use fat as a primary source of energy.) Nestled in the middle are your type IIa fibers. Scientists call these fibers fast-twitch/oxidative-glycolytic fibers. These fibers have an intermediate contraction speed, but what's most interesting is that training can make these type IIa fibers act more like type I fibers, or more like type IIb fibers, depending on what kind of training you do. Of course, endurance training will make them act more like type I's, and intense strength training will make them act more like type IIb's.

Now, your type IIb's are the real powerhouses. They're the ones capable of generating the most force the fastest, but they burn out fairly quickly. Think of them as sort of the Mike Tyson of muscle fibers, minus the ear biting and incoherent tirades. They're great in the early rounds but get into trouble if activity lasts longer than a few seconds. The type IIa's, on the other hand, are moderately resistant to fatigue yet can still produce a decent amount of force. These are the fibers you rely on most heavily for activities that take between 15 seconds and 2 minutes such as middle distance running and weight training.

It's worth noting, however, that regardless of the type of activity you do, all of these fibers work on a continuum. So during strength and power activities, some slow twitch fibers are still recruited, just as fast-twitch fibers are active to a lesser extent during endurance work. It's not as if your body flips a switch and selectively recruits a specific type of muscle fiber based on its energy needs at a given time. The other thing that warrants mention here is the fact that each of us is made up of a mix of different fiber types. No one is exclusively fast- or slow-twitch. Fiber compositions vary tremendously from person to person and, in fact, muscle to muscle (see page 50).

SPARE A LITTLE CHANGE?

As mentioned earlier, type IIa fibers can take on the properties of type I or type IIb fibers based on how you train. For instance, high repetition, lighter-load training has been shown to cause type IIa fibers to take on some of the endurance properties of type I fibers. Likewise, maximal strength and power training can result in type IIa fibers behaving more like type IIb fibers. Unfortunately, any conversion of fiber types seems to be limited to the type IIa fibers, meaning that those of you with a higher proportion of type I fibers can pretty much rule out a career as an Olympic sprinter. But just because you've been shortchanged in the fast-twitch fiber department doesn't mean you're destined to be a toothpick for the rest of your life. While it's true that slow-twitch fibers have a limited potential for hypertrophy, focusing your training efforts on stimulating what fast-twitch fibers you do have can bring about significant amounts of growth.

This can effectively be achieved by concentrating mainly on heavy load, low-rep training. Of course, this means "the big three" again! Bear in mind, though, that this is going to be a major adjustment for some of you. The majority of ectomorphs who do currently lift naturally tend to gravitate toward higher-rep training protocols with relatively lighter loads. This choice is probably a result of two things. First, higher-rep protocols are usually easier for our slow-twitch friends, and because they seem to perform better with higher-rep work, they stick with it. Second, the bodybuilding approach to strength training that still reigns supreme in most gyms influences many lifters. After all, if the big guys are doing it, the skinny guys follow suit without realizing that different folks require different strokes. Regardless of the reason why most ectomorphs end up doing higher-rep work, the end result is that most don't spend enough time stimulating those muscle fibers designed for growth—the ultrapowerful fast-twitch type IIb fibers.

The reason we even bring up the whole issue of fiber type in relation to recovery is this: Different fibers have different recovery curves. Since fast-twitch fibers may take longer to recover, different individuals, based on their fiber types, may need different training protocols to optimize recovery. So what does this mean for the ectomorph? Not much. Not yet, anyway. After all, ectomorphic physiques are usually full of slow-twitch fiber types and therefore should have great recovery rates.

But remember, the only way to force growth in the hypertrophy-challenged ectomorph is to really go after those fast-twitch type IIb fibers. Furthermore, since strength training programs that are designed to hit those type IIb fibers are very taxing on the central nervous system, and ectomorphs usually have overactive nervous systems (scrawny guys are usually hyper, aren't they?), we can now see why serious strength training requires a lot of recovery—especially for the ectomorph. However, don't make the mistake of thinking that if some rest days are good, more are better. Ectomorphs need to find the balance between training enough to stimulate growth and resting enough to allow that growth to happen. Sure, it can be tricky, but we're confident that the program contained in this book will help you do just that. Actually we know it will; we just don't want to seem too cocky.

IT'S JUST A PHASE

Part of finding this balance between work and recovery involves factoring in the type of training phase you're engaged in. Let's say, for instance, that you're working on improving your muscular strength. The heavy loads you'll likely be using will place a greater demand on your central nervous system than it encounters during more-moderate-load hypertrophy training. Therefore, you'll probably need a longer break between workouts (say about 48 to 72 hours). When training for size, on the other hand, as long as you keep the overall

WHAT'S YOUR TYPE?

To help you gain a better understanding of your individual muscle fiber composition, we'd like you to first find your 1RM (1 repetition max) on the exercises listed below.

1. Barbell Squat
2. Regular Deadlift
3. Bench Press
4. Pullup (add weight if necessary)
5. Overhead Press

Once you've determined your 1RM in each of these exercises, on a separate day, attempt to perform 85 percent of that amount for as many reps as possible. To determine your probable fiber distribution, simply consult the chart below.

>> Less than five reps at 85 percent 1RM—Fast-twitch (Type IIb) dominant in that muscle group

>> Five reps at 85 percent 1RM—Mixed fiber distribution in that muscle group

>> More than five reps at 85 percent 1RM—Slow-twitch (Type I) dominant in that muscle group

Note: Those of you who are new to lifting, or who are inexperienced in doing some of these lifts, may feel anxious about attempting a 1RM by yourself. You can also obtain a fairly accurate prediction of your 1RM using a submaximal load (so long as it's 10 reps or fewer) and plugging your values into the following formula:

$$1RM = Weight\ Lifted \times (1 + (0.033 \times n))$$

where (n) = the number of reps performed

So, if you lifted 250 pounds for, say, five reps, your 1RM would be

$$1RM = 250 \times (1 + (0.033 \times 5))$$

To do this calculation properly, you need to start by multiplying 0.033×5, and you'll get 0.165. Next, you add 1 to get 1.165. Then, you multiply 1.165×250, and you'll get 291 pounds. That's your 1RM.

For those of you who are mathematically challenged yet have access to the Internet, you can also do an online search for the Brzycki 1RM calculator, and simply plug in your numbers to obtain the value.

LIGHT MEN CAN'T JUMP?

Another great way to assess overall muscle fiber composition is a simple vertical jump test. For this test, all you'll need is a high wall, some colored chalk, a tape measure, and either a ladder or a step stool depending on how explosive you are.

Begin by marking your fingertips with the chalk and standing with your dominant side facing the wall. Next, reach your arm up straight over your head, and once you've reached as high as you can, mark the wall with your fingertips. Now, step away from the wall about 6 inches or so, and in one rapid motion, bend your knees, swing your arms back, and then explode up as high as you can. At the apex or peak of your jump, lightly touch your fingertips to the wall.

training volume within reason (more on this in a moment), and you ensure that your energy intake is adequate, lifting as frequently as four times per week can produce some impressive results. This is because your nervous system doesn't take quite the beating during this type of phase.

We realize this information may fly in the face of some conventional hardgainer wisdom, especially since we're suggesting that the hypertrophy-challenged work out more than 2 days per week, but as you've probably noticed by now, we're not afraid to challenge the current dogma, especially when we know we're right. The fact is; training frequency, should be governed by the intensity and

You then simply measure the distance between the two marks. Based on your jump height, use the following chart to determine the predominant muscle fiber type in your lower body:

» 12 to 18 inches: Slow-twitch (type I) dominant
» 18 to 24 inches: Mixed fiber distribution
» More than 24 inches: Fast-twitch (type IIb) dominant

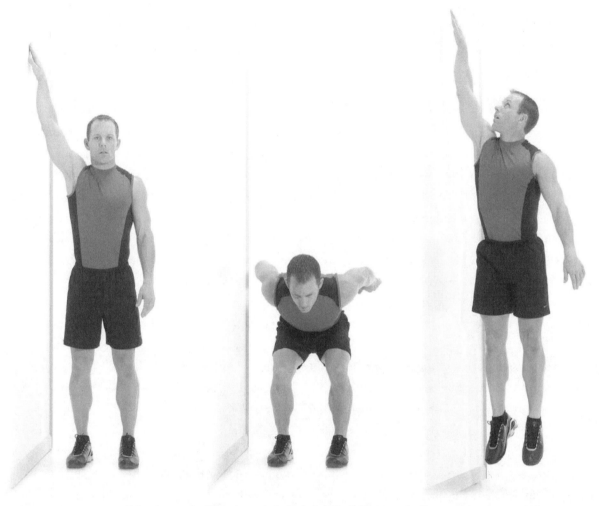

Take the vertical jump test to help determine your muscle fiber type.

volume of your workouts and not some rigid guidelines that have no sound physiological reasoning behind them.

Of course, those previous two examples we gave might give you the impression that training for size and strength are mutually exclusive. That's not the case at all. Rather, when your goal is increasing the maximal amount of weight you can lift, you'll certainly be growing! And likewise, when training to get bigger, you'll also be getting stronger. The only reason we speak in terms of "strength" programs and "hypertrophy" programs is that these descriptors address the intention of the phase, not the sole result. And with different intentions come variations in the amount of weight lifted, the repetition range used, and the amount of rest taken between sets. It only makes sense that when these variables are manipulated, things such as food intake and workout frequency need to be manipulated also. Although we'd like to tell you that forcing stubborn muscles to grow is an easy process, it's not. Fortunately for you, the training program in this book was specifically developed to account for all the variables discussed above.

TURN THAT DOWN, WILL YA?

In weight-training parlance, the term "volume" refers to the overall amount of work being done per a given unit of time. Notice, we didn't say amount of weight being lifted. You see, the amount of weight being lifted is considered "intensity." With respect to volume, the amount of work being done refers to the number of exercises, sets, and repetitions you do over the course of your workout.

In our experience, many trainees steer off course when it comes to selecting a consistent and appropriate volume. Instead of using scientific periodization principles (altering your training program systematically to force improvements based on the way your body adapts), most trainees buy into the "more is better" mindset, pounding their bodies into submission with set after set of exercises that overwhelm their ability to recover. Since this book is about building muscle the natural way, we're going to show you how to systematically alter your training so that you'll get phenomenal results without having to resort to drugs to compensate for your inappropriately selected workout volume.

The terms volume and intensity are also related in an interesting way—inversely. Despite what you think, you can't train long *and* hard. Even though long workouts feel hard, toward the end of a long workout, your true intensity (the percent of 1RM that you're working at) is severely compromised.

Therefore, it stands to reason then that if you're regularly logging 2-hour training sessions, toward the end, you can't be working very intensely. This means that although the muscle burns and you feel fatigued, you probably didn't train hard enough to stimulate those IIb fibers.

Plus, as volume goes up, those marathon training sessions create an unfavorable hormonal environment for building muscle. That's right. Longer workouts aren't muscle building. Short, intense (as measured by a high percentage of 1RM) training promotes the release of the all-natural muscle-building hormones such as growth hormone and testosterone. Long, drawn-out workouts have the opposite effect by releasing too much of the muscle-eating hormone cortisol. This catabolic (muscle-destroying) hormone makes its appearance during times of physical and mental stress and is public enemy number one on your quest to build size.

So now that we've given you some interesting information about volume and intensity, we're going to put some numbers behind our recommendations. Generally speaking, the heavier the load you're using, the more type IIb fibers you'll be using, and the fewer repetitions you'll be able to do. When using fewer repetitions, you're going to need a larger number of sets to receive an appreciable training effect. On the other hand, lighter loads and higher reps stimulate more of those type IIa and type I fibers. When working these fibers, you can get away with fewer sets. But remember, ectomorphs should focus more on the type IIb fibers.

In terms of the number of exercises you should do, during phases that use total-body routines, anywhere from three to five exercises is usually plenty, especially when the routine is comprised of the high-efficiency, neurally demanding compound lifts. When doing split routines such as the ones featured in phase IV (see Chapter 5), one or two big compound movements and possibly one isolation exer-

THE VOLUME AND INTENSITY OF TRAINING

PHASE OF TRAINING	# OF EXERCISES (PER WORKOUT)	# OF SETS (PER EXERCISE)	# OF REPS (PER SET)	REST INTERVAL BETWEEN SETS
Corrective	6–8	1–2	12–15	30 seconds
Adaptive Hypertrophy	3–5	2–4	5–8	90 seconds
Strength	2–3	3–6	2–4	3–4 minutes
Advanced Hypertrophy	4–6	2–3	6–10	2 minutes

cise should be plenty for your larger muscle groups. Smaller muscles will do better with a single exercise. The accompanying chart will help better illustrate how to manipulate training volume.

A WEIGHTY ISSUE

We could probably go on about things like central nervous system recovery and optimal rest between sets for hours. Science geeks like us will do that from time to time; it's just our nature. However, we're also weight lifters, and that side of our brain tells us that you're looking for some straightforward program solutions. Above, we offered a chart with some of the program design variables. Now, we're going to discuss optimal loading, namely, how much weight you have to lift to get bigger.

The truth is, in all of its simplicity, in order to get big, you've got to lift big and eat big. How big is big? Well, that's highly individual. But in our experience, lifting big means lifting a lot more weight than you're lifting now. Although we can't possibly know how much you're lifting now, almost all trainees we encounter underestimate their strength potential and, in doing so, fail to lift as heavy as they truly can. The human body has a remarkable capacity for generating force; just look at the granny who lifts the car up to save her grandchild. So don't sell yourself short. Lift more weight (as long as your form doesn't start getting so bad that you're risking injury).

Remember, though, while heavier loading is important, progressive loading is the real key to reaching your full physical potential. Nowadays, somewhere along the way, the message of progressive overload has been lost. Have you ever heard the story of Milon, the famous Olympian who supposedly developed his massive physical strength by picking up a calf and carrying it every day as it grew into a bull? This is the classic story of progressive overload, and regardless of whether it's true or not, it illustrates the very best way to get bigger: Lift a little more each time you train.

How has this message been lost? Well, part of the blame probably lies at the feet of the magazine publishers who regularly feature articles on various ways to "intensify" workouts including supersets, drop sets, forced negatives, and the like. While these techniques can have their place, regularly "mixing up" your training by randomly adding and subtracting these techniques from your program prevents systematic increases in the load you're lifting. Simply stated, your workouts must be progressive and systematic, or you'll never gain the muscle that you so desire. Whether this progression means lifting more weight from one workout to the next, or doing more reps with the same weight, you must in some way push your body to do more than it did the last time you trained.

Forget doing drop sets on the leg extension, or super-setting three different exercises for your chest. If you can add 50 to 100 pounds to your squat over the course of several months or even years, you're going to become a lot bigger and stronger. It's really that simple. More weight on the bar equals more muscle on your body. It doesn't even have to be a lot more weight at first. The poundage increases could be as small as 4 to 5 percent per week, perhaps even less depending on the type of lift. For instance, 5 percent of an 80-pound barbell curl is 4 pounds, but 5 percent of a 250-pound deadlift is 12.5 pounds. So you'd probably be better off being a little more aggressive when increasing the weight on compound lifts and a bit more conservative with isolation exercises. In fact, you may very well find that in some cases, the weight increments need to be as small as 1 to 2 percent per week to allow for continued progression. We know it doesn't sound like much, but over time, this can result in some huge increases. So don't be too macho to add those 1.25-pound weights to the bar each week. They might not seem like much today, but in 2 months, that's an additional 20 pounds added to your lift.

HEARTFELT CONCERNS

Now that we've addressed volume and intensity for the weight-training portion of your workout, the issue of whether or not you should do any cardiovascular/aerobic training may arise. The issue of cardiovascular training and its place in the program of the hardgainer, ectomorph, hypertrophy-challenged (take your pick) is such a point of contention that we've devoted an entire upcoming chapter to it. Although we'll delve much deeper into all the physiology shortly, we have a couple of points to address here as they pertain to training frequency.

When increasing muscle mass is the goal, ectomorphs and cardiovascular/aerobic training are about as good a fit as Jessica Simpson and Albert Einstein. When you're all ramped up on NEAT and, as a result, fidget like the Tasmanian devil on speed, the last thing you need to do is burn up precious calories you could be using for muscle building. But don't forget, your heart is the single most important muscle in your body. So what are you to do?

Well, the heart doesn't need as much work as most people think. So the addition of a little bit of cardiovascular/aerobic work is okay as long as you eat enough food to cover the added energy expenditure. After all, the amount of "cardio" we'll recommend in this book isn't much. It's not as if you're running repeated 10-K races. If you do, then you can probably forget about putting any serious strain on those shirtsleeves. But if all we're talking about is a couple of 15-minute sessions per week, don't sweat it. Follow our program, and you'll be able to pump up your pecs and your heart. In the next chapter, we'll explain how.

AR *REST* ED DEVELOPMENT

Now that we've discussed the appropriate training volumes and intensities for both strength and cardiovascular/aerobic work, it's time to discuss the rest component of recovery. We'd certainly be remiss if we didn't mention the importance of getting a good night's sleep.

If you're really serious about building up your body, getting enough sleep is going to have to be right up near the top of your priority list. Although there hasn't been much investigation into the negative effects of sleep deprivation on strength performance, at least one study demonstrated impaired motor ability and decreases in anaerobic (sprint-type) performance due to a lack of sleep.

Missing out on sleep also creates a physiological stress that is amplified when training intensely. Don't sleep enough when training heavily, and the central nervous system won't be too happy. You'll get that "tired but wired" feeling characteristic of being overworked. However, it's usually not over-work that creates the problem; it's under-rest. Unfortunately, this is usually also accompanied by a decrease in immune function. Seeing as how you can't train when you're sick, do yourself a favor, and make sure you get enough shut-eye.

Most authors suggest 8 hours per night, but sleep requirements are highly individual. We suggest getting anywhere from 6 to 9 hours of sleep per night. Your body will give you clues about whether you're getting too much or not enough.

IT'S ALL ABOUT YOU

In reading through this chapter, we hope one theme emerges: The amount of physical training your body can withstand and adapt to is dependent on a variety of factors, and only you can perfect these variables to produce the best results. Don't get suckered into thinking you have to follow some stringent, universal guidelines to get the most out of your workouts. Not even the excellent workouts presented in this book will be perfect for everyone. To get a truly perfect plan, you'll have to come see us in person or visit us at www.scrawnytobrawny.com. But as long as you keep your workouts brief and intense, and make sure you're properly rested and fueled, you *will* make gains. Just realize going in that it's not as simple as eating more and training less often than other people. There's way more to it than that.

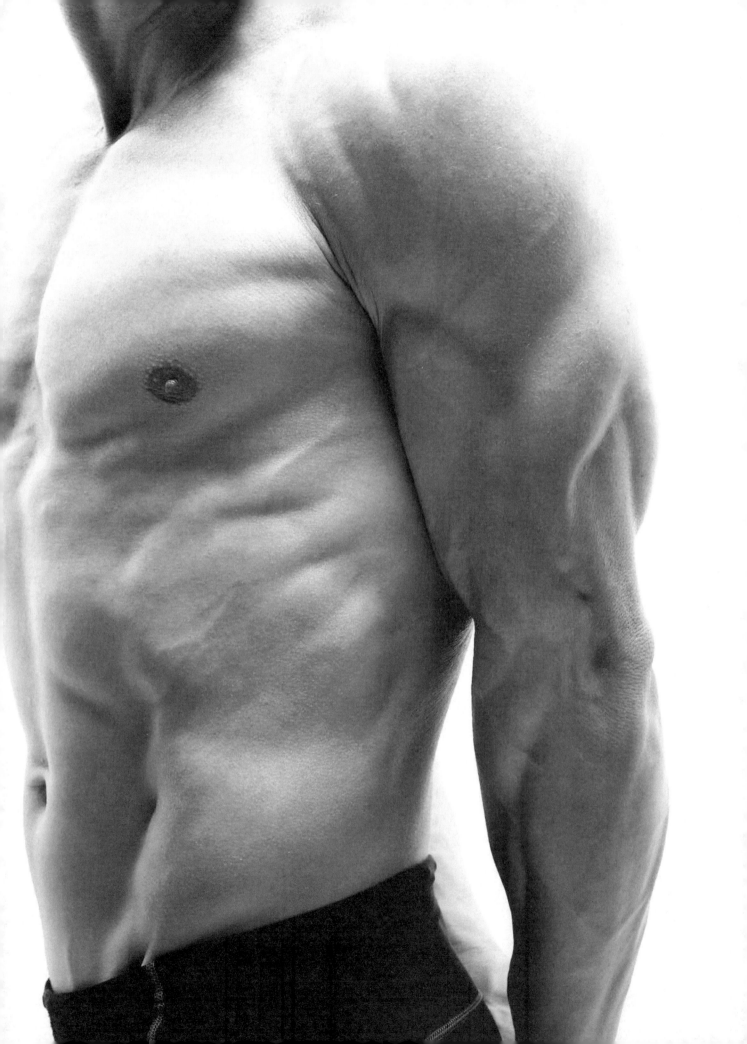

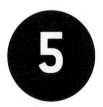

HAVE A HEART

>> Okay, we'll admit it; we're a couple of muscle heads. We much prefer the feeling of nailing a new personal best, or getting an incredible pump to the one we get from running a 5-K or doing half an hour on the elliptical machine. Call us crazy, but we never cared much for the whole runner's high, preferring instead to create our endorphin release as the result of moving heavy objects repeatedly. That said, we're also both fitness professionals and appreciate the importance of regular cardiovascular conditioning. After all, what good is it to have all those purty muscles if you need to stop for oxygen just running down the block?

When you're an ectomorph, it's important to find a balance between relaxing, saving up your energy for your weight-training workouts, and working the old ticker. To hear some experts tell it, guys who have a tough time building muscle have no business doing cardiovascular exercise. Citing the fact that cardiovascular/aerobic work expends too much energy, they argue that doing cardio will have a negative impact on one's ability to build muscle. And to a certain extent, they're right.

Too much cardio will, without question, hamper your ability to add muscle. Resistance training and traditional cardiovascular (a.k.a. aerobic) exercise are at opposite ends of the spectrum in terms of the adaptations they bring about. Therefore, doing a high volume of both will only keep you from accomplishing your goals.

But we're just not comfortable avoiding cardiovascular exercise entirely in the name of bigger biceps. Of course, certain types of resistance training do offer a decent cardiovascular stimulus. But for the most part, the type of training you'll be doing in this program does not. This heavy-load, low-rep training with relatively long rest intervals doesn't provide the same cardiovascular benefit as more continuous forms of exercise.

Don't get us wrong; your heart's still working. It's just that any elevations in heart rate are the function of constricted blood vessels in the muscles, creating an increased peripheral resistance and a bigger "roadblock" for the heart to pump against.

So in our view, it's not so much an issue of whether or not you *should* do cardio, but rather *how much* and *what type* best suits your needs. Remember, unlike the majority of folks you see draped all over the stairclimber at the local sweat palace, burning fat is the least of your problems. Your main interest in doing cardio should be for the health-related benefits. As such, your cardio workouts need to be far more intense and shorter in duration than that of the average gym rat, just like your weight training workouts. Forget the obligatory 30 to 45 minutes in the "fat-burning zone." Your workouts are going to be short and sweet. Why? Because anything more than that would likely sabotage your progress.

THE ODD COUPLE

As we alluded to earlier, resistance training and traditional aerobic exercise are incompatible at high volumes. You simply can't excel at both simultaneously. That's why you don't see a lot of bodybuilders doing triathlons, or marathon runners putting up impressive poundages in the squat rack. You can, however, engage in both to varying degrees depending on what it is you're trying to accomplish. Let us tell you how.

When building muscle is the goal, cardio needs to be kept to a minimum, especially when you have to fight for every ounce of muscle you gain. Besides, a couple of brief, intense workouts per week are really all you need to maintain good cardiovascular health. Any more than that, and you're either using cardio as a form of weight control or as a means of training for an endurance-based sport.

However, before you go ahead and just randomly start adding cardio to your program, there are a few things you need to keep in mind. First and foremost, the caloric support needs to be there. What we mean by that is that you have to make sure you eat enough calories to cover the energy demands of the workout. This shouldn't be too difficult since the workouts are going to be relatively brief (12 to 16 minutes in du-

ration, tops). The chart on the opposite page will give you the energy requirements for several different types of activities and can help you determine how many calories you need to replace based on the duration and intensity of your workouts.

The second consideration is the phase of training that you're in. During periods where you're working with lighter loads and higher reps (like Phase I), or supersets with shorter rest intervals (like Phase IV), you're probably better off doing as little cardio as possible (perhaps as few as one session per week). On the other hand, heavy-load, low-rep training, such as the type featured in Phases II and III, may have you feeling that you need a little bit more. Two short workouts per week are all you should really be doing when trying to add muscle. Otherwise, you'll just be spinning your wheels.

Finally, you need to try to keep your cardio training as far removed from your lifting as possible. We realize this might not always present the best option from a time efficiency standpoint. After all, if you can only get to the gym three times per week, it makes perfect sense to do it all in one shot. Unfortunately, though, what suits your schedule may not be optimal for building muscle. Combining resistance and cardiovascular training in the same session will likely lengthen your workouts to the point where they have a negative impact on your ability to recover. Let's face it; following a grueling session with the weights with 20 minutes on the elliptical machine isn't exactly a recipe for getting huge. Your muscles need a little more time than that to recuperate, especially considering the intense nature of the type of cardio work we want you to do.

THE HIIT PARADE

It's called HIIT (High Intensity Interval Training), and although there are lots of ways you can do it, the basic premise involves interspersing short bouts of intense activity with active recovery periods. So after a thorough warmup, you might

CALORIC COST OF VARIOUS MODES OF EXERCISE

TYPE OF ACTIVITY	METS*	KCAL/HOUR (FOR 154-LB PERSON)
High-impact aerobics	7.0	514.5
Low-impact aerobics	5.0	367.5
High-intensity cycling	12.0	882.0
Low-intensity cycling	3.0	220.5
High-intensity walking	6.5	477.8
Low-intensity walking	2.5	183.8
High-intensity running	18.0	1323.0
Low-intensity running	7.0	514.5
Circuit-type training	8.0	588.0
Intense free-weight lifting	6.0	441.0
Moderate machine training	3.0	220.5
Swimming, fast	10.0	735.0
Swimming, moderate	8.0	588.0
Jumping rope, fast	12.0	882.0
Jumping rope, medium	10.0	735.0
Jumping rope, slow	8.0	588.0
Rowing, fast	12.0	882.0
Rowing, moderate	7.0	514.5
Rowing, slow	3.5	257.0

* Metabolic equivalency unit (see page 177)

sprint for 30 seconds, then rest for 90 seconds (a light jog or brisk walk should do it). You would then repeat this sequence for the desired number of intervals, usually six to eight per workout.

With this type of training, you can get fantastic cardiovascular benefits with only 16 minutes of total exercise time (eight reps × 2 minutes per rep) or 4 minutes of actual high-intensity exercise (eight reps × 30 seconds). Another benefit of this type of training is that it allows you to do a greater percentage of the workout at a level of intensity that you wouldn't have been able to maintain had you attempted to do it continuously. Remember, intensity and duration are inversely proportional. As duration increases, intensity goes down. That's

why these HIIT workouts work so well. You do short-duration, high-intensity work, rest, and then do it again.

Another thing we really like about HIIT is that it gives you an awesome cardiovascular workout while keeping your overall energy demand fairly low. Granted, it's not the kind of typical steady pace "aerobic" work that most people have come to associate with good health, but where is it written that an exercise has to be aerobic to offer cardiovascular benefit? Things such as lowering your blood pressure, keeping your cholesterol in check, and improving overall cardiovascular efficiency are all attainable with high-intensity exercise.

Below, you'll find three different HIIT workouts

designed to best complement the type of workouts you'll find in the different weight-training phases. We've even gone so far as to select the mode of exercise that best fits the goals of a particular phase of training (although we do suggest alternatives in case you don't have access to our selections).

In Phase I, for instance, in keeping with the corrective nature of the program and heavy upper-back emphasis, we've selected rowing. In Phases II and III, though, we picked sprinting and rope jumping because of the added intensity they bring. Then in Phase IV, in addition to the mode of exercise, we also change the duration of the work and rest intervals as well as recommend a reduced training frequency to best coexist with the increased lifting volume. The end result is a custom-tailored cardio program geared toward supporting, and not impeding, your efforts in the weight room.

PHASE I CARDIO (TWO HIIT SESSIONS PER WEEK)

》 SESSION #1

Mode of exercise: Rowing (alternative: elliptical machine)

Total duration: 15 minutes (15 full intervals)

Work-to-recovery ratio: 1:3 (15 seconds work: 45 seconds recovery)

》 SESSION #2

Mode of exercise: Rowing (alternative: elliptical machine)

Total duration: 16–20 minutes (8–10 full intervals)

Work-to-recovery ratio: 1:3 (30 seconds work; 90 seconds recovery)

PHASE II & III CARDIO (TWO HIIT SESSIONS PER WEEK)

》 SESSION #1

Mode of exercise: Sprinting or jumping rope (alternative: swimming)

Total duration: 16 minutes (8 full intervals)

Work-to-recovery ratio: 1:3 (30 seconds work; 90 seconds recovery)

》 SESSION #2

Mode of exercise: Sprinting or jumping rope (alternative: swimming)

Total duration: 15 minutes (5 full intervals)

Work-to-recovery ratio: 1:3 (45 seconds work; 135 seconds recovery)

PHASE IV CARDIO (2 HIIT SESSIONS PER WEEK*)

》 SESSION #1

Mode of exercise: Stairclimbing (alternative: cycling)

Total duration: 16 minutes (8 full intervals)

Work-to-recovery ratio: 1:3 (30 seconds work; 90 seconds recovery)

》 SESSION #2

Mode of exercise: Stairclimbing (alternative: cycling)

Total duration: 16 minutes (4 full intervals)

Work-to-recovery ratio: 1:3 (60 seconds work; 180 seconds recovery)

In some instances, once a week may suffice.

GAUGING INTENSITY

Since we're not necessarily going to ask you to monitor your heart rate to determine how hard you're working, we need to come up with some other way to gauge your intensity during both the work and recovery phases of each interval. One easy way to do this is to use a scale of 1 to 10 to rate how hard you feel you're working. Working with the assumption that 10 represents your maximal effort (in other words, 10 means you could only go at this intensity for a few brutal seconds before being embarrassingly shot off the treadmill), we want you to choose the following work and rest intensities.

Sure, this is somewhat less scientific than heart-rate measures, but unless you've got one of those fancy heart-rate monitors, it's about the only practical way to gauge intensity when you're doing some of these workouts. Try putting two fingers to the side of your neck and counting while you're jumping rope, or better yet, sprinting. Trust us, it's not gonna happen. Besides, for some of the short-duration work, the heart rate will rise throughout the work interval. So you won't be able to pin down what intensity you're at anyway.

Another way to gauge intensity is to adjust the level of work (i.e., most gym equipment allows you to alter the level of intensity according to some numeric scale) for each interval. For example, we might have

an individual do cycle sprints at the machine's designated "level 10" for 30 seconds at a fast cadence (more than 120 rpm) and then reduce the level to "3" for 90 seconds. Different machines have different measures, however. Rowing machines, for example, don't offer different levels but do offer watt output designations and time per 500-meter designations. In using the rower, someone might row at a 1:50/500 meter pace for 30 seconds, and a 2:20/500 meter pace for 90 seconds. Alternatively, he might row at 200W [WATTS] for 30 seconds and 130W for 90 seconds. And, of course, on a treadmill, you've got speed. A typical person may run at 10 mph for 60 seconds and walk at 4 mph for 180 seconds.

Remember, though, these are just examples of how to gauge intensity in the gym. Some of you may choose to swim, bike, or run outdoors. That's fine, too. Just be sure that you're choosing the appropriate intensity for your efforts. Most people far underestimate their ability when doing intervals, so when they call a particular workout a "9" according to our perceived effort scale above, it's really just a "5." How could they be so off? Simply put, they haven't ever worked at a "10," so they have no basis for ranking. Seriously, assume that a "10" is represented by your running from a rabid grizzly, and you'll have a good comparison point.

WORK AND REST DURATION (SECONDS)	WORK AND REST INTENSITY RATINGS (FROM 1–10)
15 : 45	9.5 : 3
30 : 90	9 : 4
45 : 135	8.5 : 5
60 : 180	8 : 5

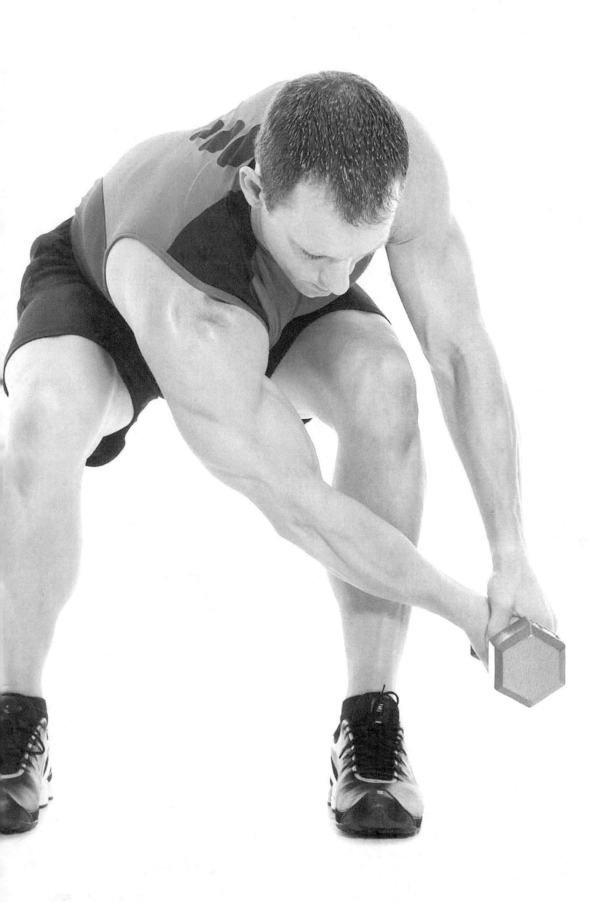

TRAINING: PHASE I

Finally, it's time to start putting together the workout! It's time to take all of the information we've discussed in the previous few chapters and use it for what it was intended—to build muscle. But before we give you the keys to the car, before we unleash you on that power cage, it's time to make sure your body is ready for your enthusiasm. Because when you're pushing the heavy iron, any and all weaknesses become exposed. Either you address them now or end up paying for them down the road.

In just a few short weeks, during Phase II, you'll be throwing around some heavy weights using "the big three" as your foundation. But before you're ready to launch this assault on your skeletal muscles, tendons, and ligaments, we've got to introduce this preparatory phase of training. The preparatory phase is designed to help correct any muscle imbalances you might have developed during a prior training program. But not only incorrect training creates imbalance; even sitting in a desk chair all day can do so.

What kind of imbalances are we talking about? Things such as insufficient core strength or a pronounced difference in flexibility from one side of the body to the other can not only limit your results but, if severe enough, can serve as precursors to injury. A perfect example of this is the anterior (front) shoulder dominance commonly displayed by most men at the gym. Because of their penchant for overworking the "mirror muscles," specifically the pecs, lats, and biceps, the average trainee ends up with a visible imbalance between the muscles that act on the anterior (front) and posterior (rear) aspects of the shoulder. In the end, the anterior muscles begin to pull the shoulders forward, causing a distinct rounding of the shoulders. As a result of this imbalance, trainees with anterior dominance begin to look more like Cro-Magnon men than Homo sapiens.

Although this condition exists to varying degrees, if not addressed, it can manifest as a shoulder impingement, a painful condition where tendons and ligaments get pinched between two bony structures. You may not feel it when working with lighter loads, but continue adding weight to the bar, and sooner or later, it'll make its presence known.

Therefore this first phase is like an automobile maintenance check. You wouldn't take your car out on a long trip in hazardous road conditions without first doing some sort of maintenance check, right? So don't do the same with your body. Exercise some patience, and slowly work through our preparatory phase so that it'll be smooth driving once the overload in Phase II begins.

One of the best parts about this preparatory phase is that, based on nine simple tests below, you can individualize this phase so that you're correcting your own personal imbalances. That's right, by the end of this chapter, you'll have your very own preparatory/corrective phase designed specifically for your body. No generic programs here.

POSTURAL ASSESSMENT

As indicated, the following nine tests are going to reveal a whole lot about the way your body currently functions. But we'll warn you up front, when clients come to see us, it's usually not pretty, regardless of how advanced they think they are. But don't be embarrassed by your results. These tests are designed to uncover weak links in your body's ability to perform, not give you an ego boost. Once you've identified and corrected these weak links, your training in Phases II through IV will be that much better.

Before you get started, though, bear in mind that while some of these tests allow for easy self-assessment, others will require you to enlist the

help of a friend or training partner to observe you as you do them. Better yet, having that person videotape you performing the tests would allow you to assess yourself later.

Well, what are you waiting for? Get to work!

The Pencil Test

This one seems harmless enough, but as you'll soon find out, it can reveal a lot about what's going on at the shoulder joint. We got this test from Ken Kinakin, D.C., founder of the Society of Wellness Integrated Specialists (S.W.I.S.) and author of the excellent book *Optimal Muscle Training*. To begin, grab a couple of pencils and hold them in your hands with the points facing out and your arms at your sides. Look down at your hands. Where are the pencils pointed? If they're pointed straight ahead, and your arms are right next to your sides, you're golden; move on to the next test. But, if they're pointed inward diagonally, slightly facing the front of your thighs, give yourself 1 point. If they're pointing toward each other, so it looks like you're about to poke yourself in the jewels, give yourself 2 points.

The problem: This test is designed to assess the degree of internal rotation at the shoulder joint. Ideally, your arms should drop down right next to your sides with your palms facing each other. Oftentimes, however, things such as too much chest and lat work, tight pecs, and poor postural habits can cause the upper arms to rotate inward and pull the shoulders across the front of the body. It's that Cro-Magnon thing again. Besides being rather unattractive, this also indicates an imbalance between the muscles that internally and externally rotate the shoulder. Having weak, overstretched external rotators increases your likelihood of developing a shoulder impingement, or possibly even a rotator cuff tear.

The fix: If there is a problem, depending on the

degree to which it exists, the first strategy is to stretch the pecs, lats, front deltoids, and biceps (see Chapter 6). In addition, strengthening the muscles that externally rotate the humerus (upper arm bone) and retract the scapula can often help correct the problem. For strengthening the external rotators, this means various forms of external rotation exercises such as the ones found on pages 103, 127, and 144. For strengthening the scapula retractors, use various rowing movements with the elbows held out away from the body and an emphasis on pinching the shoulder blades together. These types of rows de-emphasize the lats (which are powerful internal rotators in their own right) by giving them a less-favorable angle of pull, thus increasing the demand on the postural muscles of the upper back.

If you gave yourself a 1 during the pencil test, along with daily stretching for those muscles that are tight, you're going to do two or three times as much work for the muscles that retract your shoulders and externally rotate your arms as you do chest and lat work. This means that exercises like various types of rows, reverse flyes, and external rotations will far outnumber the ever popular bench press and lat pulldown. Complete descriptions of all of these exercises along with recommended set and repetition schemes can be found at the end of this chapter.

If you scored a 2, brace yourself, pal. You're completely off all chest and lat training for the next few weeks. Don't worry though, your chest won't shrivel up and die. In fact, you'll probably notice a slight increase in strength once you reintroduce pec work in Phase II. This increased strength will come courtesy of the improved muscular balance that now exists at the shoulder joint. We've provided you with examples of how to do this in the sample workouts at the end of this chapter.

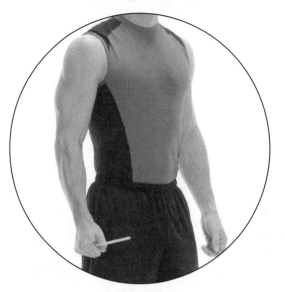

Optimal posture

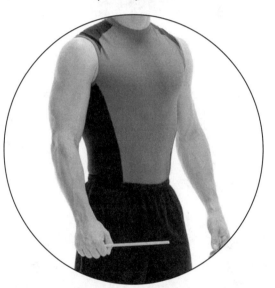

Slight internal rotation

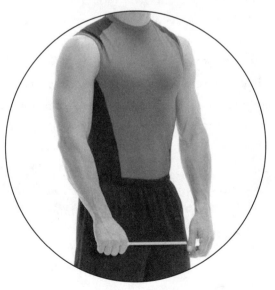

Severe internal rotation

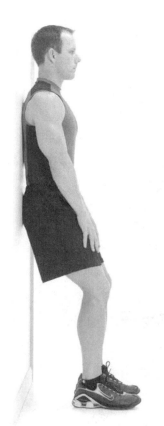
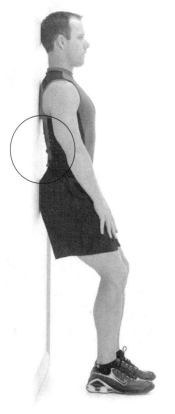
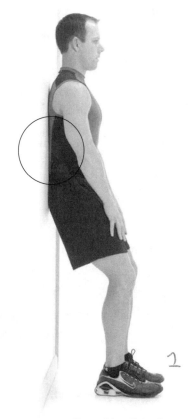

| Optimal pelvic tilt | Severe anterior tilt | Posterior pelvic tilt |

The Pelvic Tilt

Here's another simple test. Stand relaxed with your back to a wall and your feet approximately 1 foot out in front of you (measured at the heel). Make sure your rear end, shoulder blades, and the back of your head are all in contact with the wall. Next, reach one arm behind you just above the waist, and attempt to slide your hand between your lower back and the wall. If you can fit your hand (but not much more) into this space, continue on to the next test. If you can fit a fist (1 point), or worse yet, most of your forearm (2 points) between your back and the wall, your pelvis is rotated in the anterior direction. If you can't even fit your hand into this space (1 point), your pelvis is rotated in the posterior direction. These are rather common problems that are often the result of poor postural habits, tight muscles, and overworking specific muscle groups at the expense of others.

The problem: A pelvis that is rotated anteriorally indicates tight hip flexors and a weakened abdominal wall, whereas a pelvis that is rotated posteriorally indicates tight hamstrings and possibly weakened spinal erectors. Either way, if there's an issue here, you'll need some specific stretching and strengthening exercises to do to address these problems. Having a pelvis that deviates one way or the other can serve as a major obstacle to doing some of the lifts you need to pack on the muscle, to say nothing of the impact it has on your ability to move freely.

The fix: Those of you who have an anterior tilt will focus on hip flexor stretching and abdominal strengthening. If you suffer from a posterior tilt, look forward to doing lots of hamstring stretching and strengthening those spinal erectors. Examples for how much of each to do will once again be provided at the end of this chapter. Keep in mind, however, that just as the way internal rotation of the humerus varies

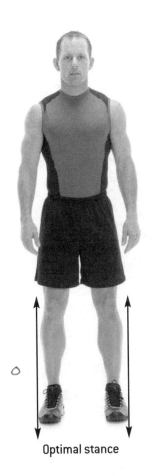
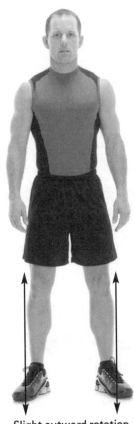
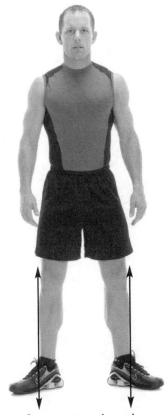

| Optimal stance | Slight outward rotation | Severe outward rotation |

in degrees of severity, so too does the degree to which the pelvis can be tilted anteriorally or posteriorly. However, because spinal mechanics are far more intricate than those of the shoulder, anything more than basic recommendations as to how to address these problems is beyond the scope of this book.

Foot Placement

This is without question the easiest one of them all. Simply stand relaxed, and look down at which way your feet are pointing. If they're pointed straight ahead, go on to the next test. If they're turned out slightly, to 11 o'clock or 1 o'clock, give yourself 1 point. If they're turned out significantly, give yourself 2 points, and seriously consider flying south for the winter.

The problem: While there are a few things that could be going on here, this is usually a combination of weak glutes (primarily the gluteus maximus)

and tightness in the Tensor Fascia latae (TFL) and iliotibial band (ITB) on the lateral part of the thigh.

When too tight, these two work together to inhibit the glutes from preventing internal rotation of the femur (upper thighs turning inward). In an effort to compensate for this internal rotation, there's usually external rotation going on at the ankle (feet turned outward) to prevent you from falling over. Keep in mind, this is sort of the *Reader's Digest* version of what's going on. You're likely also to have tight adductors (muscles that bring the legs toward the midline of the body) and weak abductors (muscles that take the leg away from the midline of the body). We just wanted to avoid another full-blown physiology lesson.

Here's an easy way to confirm if this is indeed the problem. It comes from Eric Cressey, a strength coach and graduate student at the University of Connecticut. Eric suggests the following: If you tend to

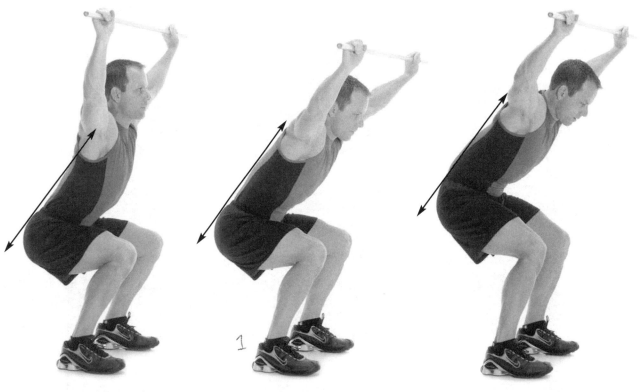

| Optimal overhead squat | Limited range overhead squat | Poor overhead squat |

stand with your feet turned out, point them straight ahead, and take a look at what's going on at the knees. Chances are they're being pulled medially (inward). Next, tighten your glutes by clenching your cheeks together. Now look at your knees again. We're willing to bet that the resulting external rotation of the femur caused them to point straight forward. Not to sound like pains in the butt, pun intended, but you've got some glute strengthening to do, mister.

The fix: In addition to strengthening the hip extensors and abductors with exercises such as the Unilateral Deadlift and Plate Drags, stretching the TFL, ITB, adductors, and hip flexors should help immensely. You'll find some great stretches for them in the flexibility section that begins on page 78.

FLEXIBILITY ASSESSMENT
Overhead Squat

To execute this drill properly requires a significant amount of flexibility around the shoulder, hip,

and ankle joints. So you needn't worry about hoisting a loaded barbell above your head and descending into a squat. For now at least, a broomstick will do just fine.

To begin, stand with your feet slightly wider than shoulder width apart and knees slightly bent, holding a broomstick at arm's length with a snatch grip (approximately twice your shoulder width). Position your feet to point either straight ahead or *slightly* out to the sides. Next, raise the bar over your head until your arms are completely straight, just out of your peripheral vision. All you have to do now is squat! That is, without allowing your arms to come forward, rounding your back, or letting your heels come off the ground. Yeah, makes it a bit tougher, doesn't it?

If you're able to descend into a full squat (backs of your thighs touching your calves) while meeting the criteria listed above, move on to the next test. If you can make it to parallel (tops of your thighs par-

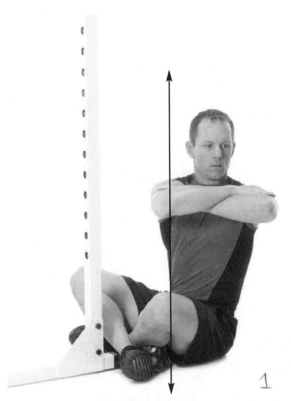

Optimal trunk rotation

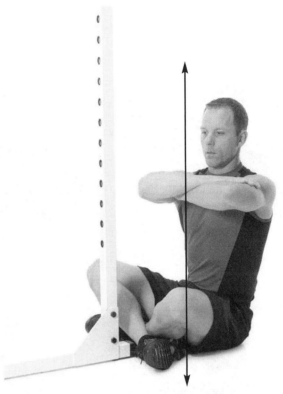

Limited range trunk rotation

allel to the floor), give yourself 1 point. If you made it halfway down (thighs and calves form a 45-degree angle), give yourself 2 points. If you barely descended an inch before various body segments started moving all over the place, you've got some serious flexibility work to do.

Areas of concentration: Hip flexors/quads, calves, chest, and shoulders. See specific stretches in Chapter 6.

Trunk Rotation

Sit on the floor in the threshold of a doorway with your legs crossed and one foot on each side of the door jam. Next, fold your arms across your body, and touch your fingertips to your shoulders as shown. Once in this position, rotate as far as you can to one side, being sure to keep your back straight and shoulder blades pinched together throughout the movement. When you've gone as far as you can, note the degree of torso

rotation by once again using our reliable clock reference. If you made it all the way, or close to 9 o'clock, go on to the next test. If you made it to 10 o'clock, give yourself one point, and if you only made it to 11 o'clock, and your trailing shoulder (right if you're turning to the left and vice versa) barely cleared the door jam, give yourself two points.

Restrictions in your ability to rotate the torso indicate tightness in the oblique muscles, specifically in the side that you're turning away from. Tightness in these muscles, especially if there's a large disparity from one side to the other, can alter your mechanics during a number of different lifts. When this happens, greater stress is incurred on one side of the body compared with the other, setting the stage for either injury or lopsided development. Needless to say, neither option is particularly attractive, especially since some targeted flexibility work can often alleviate the problem.

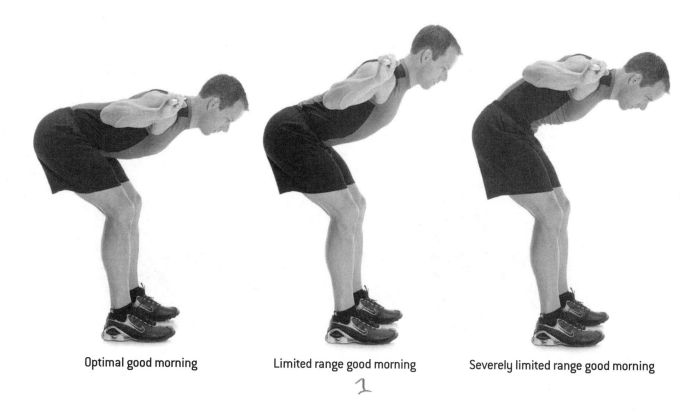

Optimal good morning   Limited range good morning   Severely limited range good morning

1

Areas of concentration: Internal and external obliques.

Arched Back Good Morning

The goal of this test is to lean forward at the waist while maintaining a slightly arched back to assess the functional flexibility of the hamstrings. What do we mean by *functional*? We're looking to assess the flexibility of your hamstrings in a position specific to the way you're going to use them during training. Sure, it's nice to lie down and pull your leg back, but that gives you information only about your static flexibility. Unfortunately, static flexibility doesn't always carry over well to dynamic movements. Seeing as how many of the lifts you're going to do are going to require you to maintain a slight lumbar lordosis (arch in the lower back), we thought this would be a more practical way to measure flexibility.

To begin, simply whip out your handy broomstick again, and rest it across your upper trapezius, as if about to perform a set of squats. Next, maintaining a slight bend in your knees, lift your chest up high to create a nice arch in your lower back. From here on, all you have to do is lean forward at the waist without allowing your back to round or your knees to straighten. Keep in mind, though, your knees shouldn't bend more either; rather just maintain the same slight 5 to 10 degrees of flexion they began the test with. If you're able to descend to the point where your torso is parallel to the floor without losing your lordosis, go on to the next test. If you can only make it about halfway down, give yourself 1 point. If you barely start to move before your back rounds or your knees straighten, give yourself 2 points.

Areas of concentration: Hamstrings.

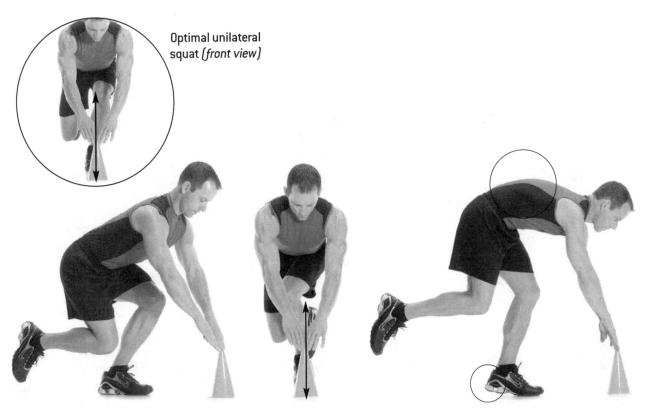

Optimal unilateral squat *(front view)*

Optimal unilateral squat *(side view)*   Unilateral squat with knee pinch   Unilateral squat with heel lift and rounded back

MUSCULAR STRENGTH ASSESSMENT
Unilateral Squat and Reach

This test can actually be used to assess a variety of things all at once. First off, it can give you a lot of information about the flexibility of your hips and calves. It can also uncover potential strength imbalances between the muscles that act on the medial (inside) and lateral (outside) aspects of the knee joint. Finally, it can also be used to see if you rely too heavily on your quads (front thigh muscles) during squatting-type movements. Besides which, it's a nice way to keep your ego in check, which makes it all the more fun to prescribe.

To begin, select an object that is no more than about 10 to 12 inches high, like a light dumbbell standing on one end or a couple of phone books stacked on top of each other. Place the object on the floor approximately 12 to 18 inches in front of you

(if you've got long arms, stay closer to 18 inches; short arms, stay closer to 12 inches), and stand on one leg by bending the non-working leg 90 degrees as shown. Here's where the fun starts: Begin to simultaneously squat down and reach forward to touch the object. In doing so, you should make sure that you're sitting back onto your heel as much as possible, and your knee is staying in line with your hip and foot. It's also okay to round your back slightly because you're not working with a heavy load; just be sure to pull your abdominals in tight toward your spine.

If you're able to descend all the way down into a parallel squat with your knee in line with your hip and foot, lightly touch the cone, stand back up, and go on to the next test. If you can get down to the bottom, but your knee either pinches in, bows out to the side, or extends well past your toes, give yourself 1 point. If you immediately start to feel

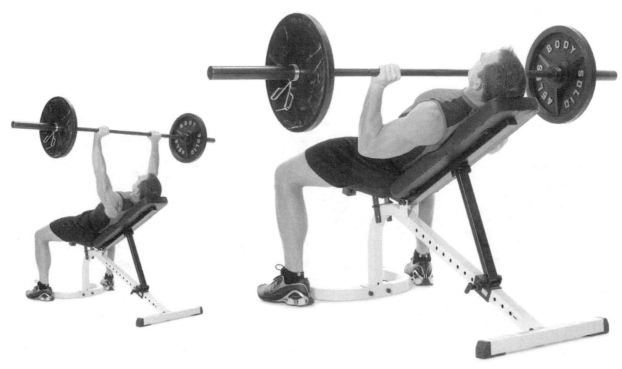

Incline bench press

your heel coming up off the floor as you descend, give yourself 2 points.

An inability to squat during this test without your heel coming off the ground signals tightness in your hip flexors and calves. Obviously, this means you've got some flexibility work to do. Assuming that you are able to get down to the required depth but you notice your knee "wandering" in places it shouldn't, you've got some strength imbalances to correct. If you see your knee shooting forward, well past your toes, and feel most of your weight on the ball of the foot, you're relying too much on your quads. The fix here is some targeted strengthening for the glutes, hamstrings, and spinal erectors, a.k.a. the "posterior chain."

Strengthening these muscles will make a dramatic difference in the loads you'll be able to handle when performing squats and deadlifts. A knee that pinches inward could possibly signal weakness in the hip abductors (muscles on the lateral aspect of the hips), or a weak VMO (vastus medialis obliquis), the innermost of the quad muscles right next to the knee. Whereas a knee that bows outward could indicate weak adductors (muscles that act on the medial aspect of the thighs). In either case, specific strengthening exercises for those areas established as weak links can often lead to tremendous improvements in knee stability. You'll see more about how to address these specific problems in the sample workouts at the end of this chapter.

Incline Bench Press/ External Rotation

This is a fantastic test we got from renowned Canadian strength coach Charles Poliquin. Having worked with some of the biggest and strongest athletes in the world, Charles knows a thing or two

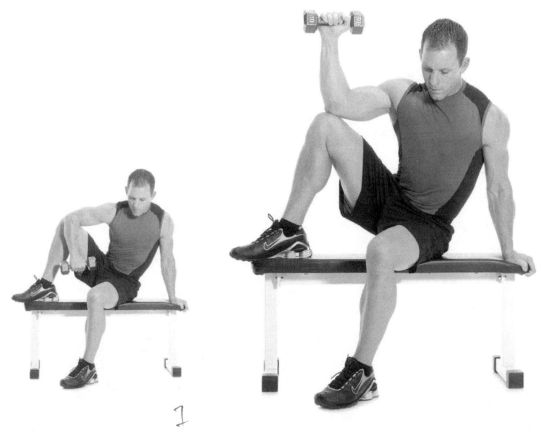

Unilateral external rotation

about proper strength ratios. And seeing how many guys fall prey to shoulder injuries brought about by poor muscular balance, we figured this would be a good test to include. The first thing you're going to need to do for this test is find your 1 repetition maximum (1RM) on the incline bench press, 1RM simply being the maximal amount of weight you can lift one time. See Chapter 4 for information about establishing your 1RM on specific lifts.

Once you've determined this value, the next thing you'll need to do is calculate 9 percent of it. So, say you had a max incline press of 200 pounds, 9 percent would be equal to 18 pounds. What this means is that you should be able to perform eight reps of the single arm external rotation exercise pictured above.

Exercise description: Sit sideways on a bench with your right foot up on the bench and your leg bent 90 degrees, and your other foot on the floor.

Holding the dumbbell in your right hand, place the inside of your right elbow on the inside of your right knee. Sitting up as straight as you can, begin with the working forearm facing down toward the floor. Using the elbow as a hinge, slowly rotate your forearm up until it is perpendicular to the floor. In doing so, be sure you don't extend your wrist back; keep your hand lined up directly over your forearm. Once at the top, pause momentarily, and then lower back to the starting position. If you were able to complete eight reps as described, go on to the next test. If you could only do a couple of reps, give yourself 1 point. If you couldn't even get the weight through the full range of motion, give yourself 2 points.

As mentioned previously, weak external rotators can place you at risk for potentially serious shoulder injuries. By de-emphasizing chest and lat work and taking the time to actively strengthen the

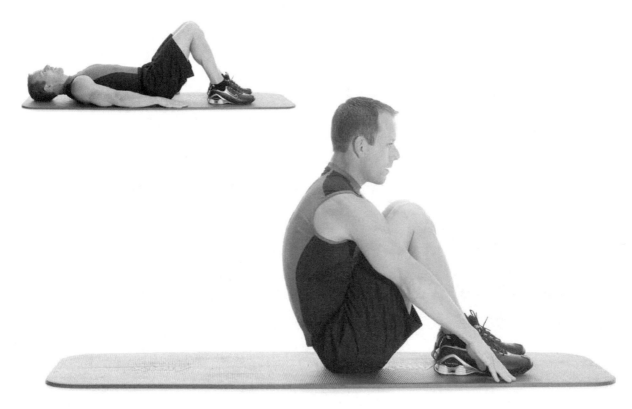

Slow situp

muscles that act on the posterior aspect of the shoulder, you may find that once you do go back to pressing exercises for the chest, your weights will actually increase due to your improved shoulder stability.

Unanchored Situp

Yeah, yeah, we know all about situps being "bad" for your back. The thing is, though, like the much-maligned squat, it isn't situps per se that are the problem; it's the way most people execute them. We freely admit that if you anchor your feet under something and jerk your head and neck forward like you've just been rear-ended, there's a good chance you'll hurt your back. But if you don't anchor your feet and are forced to come up at a significantly reduced pace, all of a sudden, the focus shifts from your back to those all-important core muscles. Unlike crunches, which "isolate" your abs

through a minuscule range of motion, situps require you to use your abdominals, hip flexors, and spinal erectors as one functional unit, the way you do in real life.

To begin, lie on your back with your knees bent approximately 90 degrees and your feet flat on the floor. Keeping your arms down at your sides, begin by slowly rolling your torso up toward your thighs, taking a full 5 seconds to reach the top position. Once there, pause for a second, and take another 5 seconds to lower yourself back. Be sure not to use any momentum by thrusting your arms forward on the way up; keep your fingers sliding along the floor the whole way up. You also have to keep your feet glued to the floor throughout the exercise. If you can complete the exercise as shown, go on to the next test. If you made it up, but your feet came up ever so slightly off the floor, give yourself 1 point. If you barely got your shoulder blades off the ground before your abs "locked up" and you had to stop, give yourself 2 points.

The ability to sit all the way up at this slow speed without anchoring your feet under something challenges your core musculature in a manner much different than most abdominal exercises. It requires you to activate your TVA (transverse abdominis), the deepest and arguably most important of your abdominal muscles. This corset-like muscle helps increase spinal stability, yet despite its importance, goes largely ignored in most abdominal training programs. The other thing the full situp does is force your abdominals to work through a much larger range of motion than the overused crunch. Seeing how few of the movements you make in daily life will require an isolated contraction of the abs through such a short range of motion, full situps have far more functional value.

THE FINAL TALLY

Now that all the numbers are in, add up your score from the preceding tests, and compare your total to the numbers listed below:

)) 0 to 5 points: Your body is in pretty good working order. A 2- to 3-week corrective phase with some focused flexibility work will probably have you adequately prepared for the program.

)) 6 to 12 points: You've got some work to do. You'll likely need a full 4-week corrective phase before getting into the more intensive training that starts in Phase II.

)) 13 points and up: You're an accident waiting to happen. Jump right into the teeth of this program without going through the corrective phase, and we can practically guarantee that you'll end up hurt. In addition to a full 4-week (if

not 6-week) corrective phase and intensive daily flexibility work, you can count on including some weak-link strengthening well into the subsequent phases.

Bear in mind that these scores are very subjective. Most of you simply don't have the experience that we do in spotting some of these conditions, so your numbers might be a bit off. They will at least, however, give you some idea of where your weak links lie. Once you're armed with this information, all you need to do is incorporate some of the exercises and stretches we've provided in this chapter, and before long, you'll be seeing marked improvements in performance. Before we get started, though, there are two things that warrant further mention:

1. Because everyone has different weaknesses/imbalances, it doesn't make sense to just include generic workouts in this section (although we will provide you with a couple of examples based on different scenarios). Instead, what we'll do is show you how to select which exercises to do from a template. You then simply choose which drills to include based on where your weaknesses lie. This makes your program highly individualized.

2. As you may have noticed in compiling your results, you may have written different scores for each limb on a particular test. For instance, during the pencil test, you may have noticed that your left arm rotates inward more than your right. Or that during the squat and reach, one leg did the test just fine, while the other had a few issues. All you have to do in this instance is include an extra set or two of strengthening, or more stretching, for whichever side is lagging behind.

SELF-ASSESSMENT SCORE SHEET

POSTURAL ASSESSMENT

The Pencil Test: R __1__ / L __1__

The Pelvic Tilt: _____1_____

Foot Placement: R __0__ / L __0__

FLEXIBILITY ASSESSMENT

Overhead Squat: _____1_____

Trunk Rotation: R __1__ / L __1__

Arched Back Good Morning: _____1_____

MUSCULAR STRENGTH ASSESSMENT

Unilateral Squat and Reach: R __1__ / L __1__

Incline Bench Press/External Rotation: R __1__ / L __1__

Unanchored Situp: _____0_____

TOTAL: _____11_____

IT'S A S-T-R-E-T-C-H

Okay, so maybe you don't stretch as often as you should. In fact, judging from some of your scores, maybe you don't stretch at all. No problem. After all, it's never too late to get started. You're going to be completely changing the way you train and eat anyway, so you might as well make it three for three. The thing is, though, we don't just want you to stretch for the sake of stretching; there's a certain way we want you to go about it.

Prior to your workouts, we want you to focus primarily on dynamic stretches, or stretches that are done while your body is in motion. After your workouts, or on off days from training, you'll do static stretching. Static stretching is the kind of stretching that most people are accustomed to. It's the type of stretching where you a hold a muscle in the stretched position for 15 to 30 seconds at a time.

The reason why we suggest dynamic stretching before workouts and static stretching after is because static stretching has been shown to lead to decrements in strength and power production when done immediately prior to strength training. Since dynamic stretching can actually improve your training session, that's the one you'll be doing prior to exercise.

In this chapter, what we've done is provide you with an array of static and dynamic stretches to choose from. Depending on where you're tight and what muscle groups you'll be training, you'll likely opt for certain stretches over others. We've also given you a couple of examples about how to best group these stretches prior to your workout.

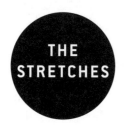

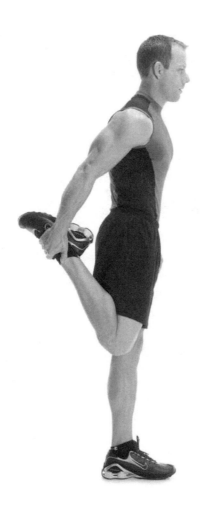

Quad Stretch Walk

(quads)

From a standing position, grab your right instep, and pull your heel toward your butt. Hold for a second; then take a step, and do the same with the other leg. Continue this way until you've covered the desired distance.

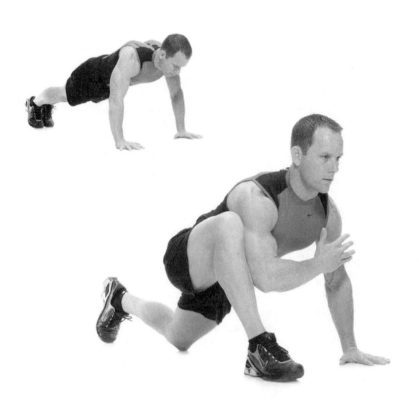

Spidermans

(hip flexors, quads, adductors)

In a pushup position, pick up your right foot, and bring it around until it plants softly right next to your right hand. Simultaneously pick up your right hand, and drop your right forearm toward the floor perpendicular to your shin. As you do so, drop your left hip and knee toward the floor. Bring your leg back, and repeat to the other side.

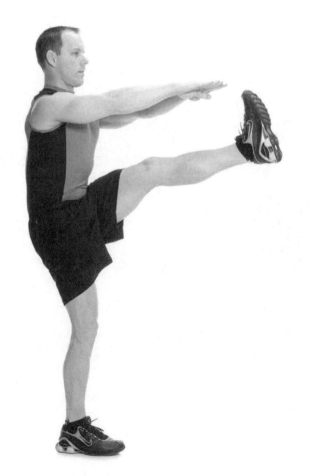

Frankensteins

(hamstrings)

With arms held out in front of you, kick your leg straight up toward your hands without dropping your chest or rounding your back. Repeat with your other leg, and continue for the desired number of reps.

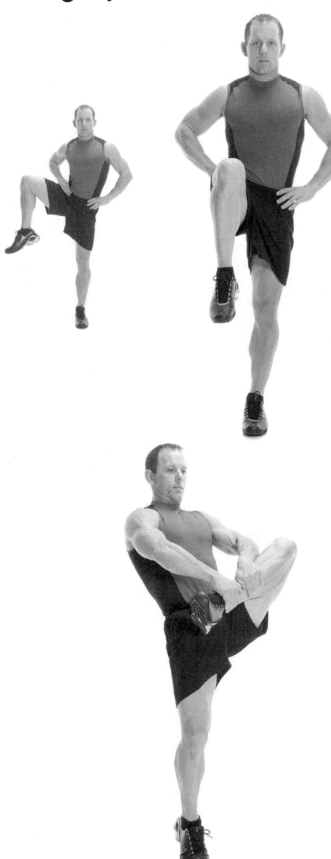

Gate Swings
(adductors)

From a standing position, lift your right knee out to the side until it's just above your belt line. Once there, swing your leg around in front of you, and lower it forward as you repeat the same sequence with the other leg.

Hip Walks
(glutes)

From a standing position, lift your right leg across the front of your body, and grab your right shin. Once you have it, simultaneously pull up, so the shin ends up parallel to the floor, and you come up on the ball of your back foot. Lower, step forward, and repeat with the other leg.

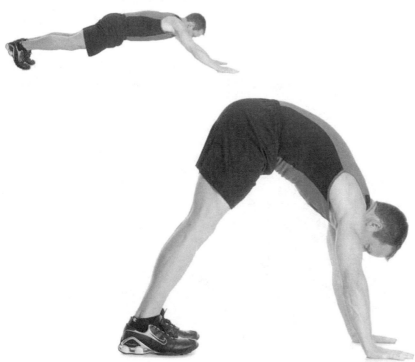

Pike Walks
(calves, hamstrings/abs, hip flexors)

From a pushup position, walk your hands forward, so they're well in front of your head. Keeping your legs totally straight, start walking your feet toward your hands. Once you've gotten as close as you can, slowly walk your hands back out to the starting position.

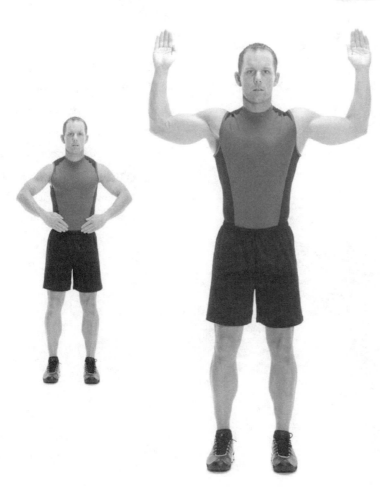

Traffic Cop
(external/internal rotators)

From a standing position, lift your arms out to the sides like a scarecrow with your arms bent 90 degrees. Starting with your forearms perpendicular to the floor, rotate your arms at the shoulder, so your hands point toward the floor. Pause, and bring them back up, making sure not to change the amount of bend in your elbows.

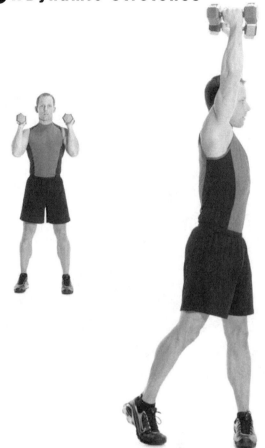

Rotational Overhead Press
(obliques, lats)

From a standing position, hold a pair of light dumbbells even with your ears. Simultaneously press them overhead, and rotate to one side. Lower them back down, and repeat to the other side.

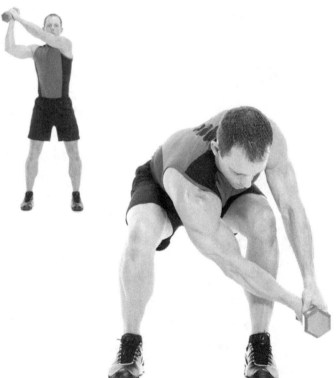

Slow Wood Chop
(obliques, lower back)

From a standing position, hold a light medicine ball or dumbbell (5 to 7 pounds) with both arms extended over your right shoulder. In one sweeping motion, slowly chop it down and across your body, finishing with your hands even with your left calf. Raise, and repeat.

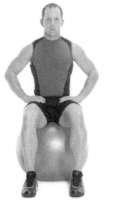
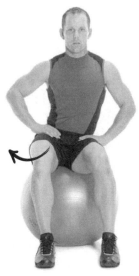
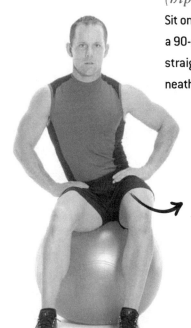

Swiss Ball Figure 8s

(hips, lower back)

Sit on a Swiss Ball, so your knees form a 90-degree angle. Keeping your torso straight and tall, roll your hips underneath you in a figure-8 pattern.

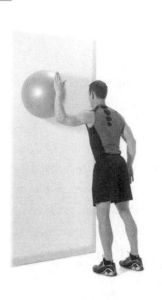
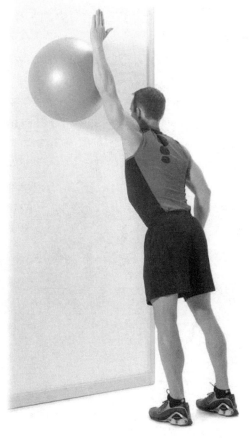

Swiss Ball Wall Rolls

(lats, shoulders)

Stand facing a wall. Place the Swiss Ball up on the wall to your left side, even with your shoulder. With your left arm bent on the ball at a 90-degree angle, simultaneously straighten your arm by rolling the ball up the wall and leaning into it. Repeat with right arm.

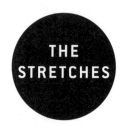

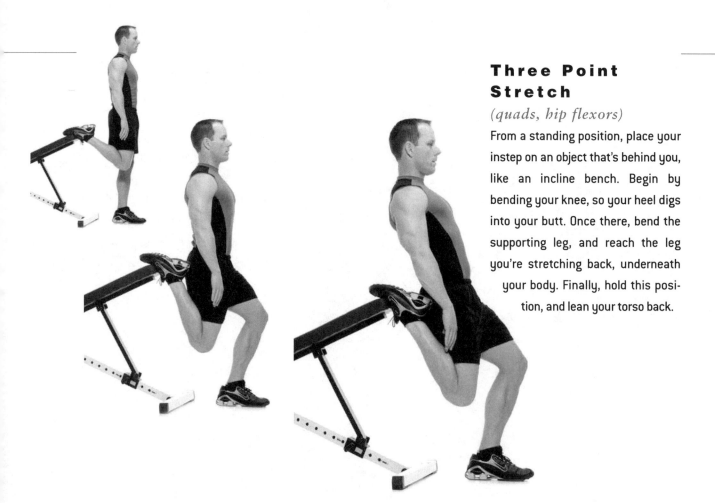

Three Point Stretch

(quads, hip flexors)

From a standing position, place your instep on an object that's behind you, like an incline bench. Begin by bending your knee, so your heel digs into your butt. Once there, bend the supporting leg, and reach the leg you're stretching back, underneath your body. Finally, hold this position, and lean your torso back.

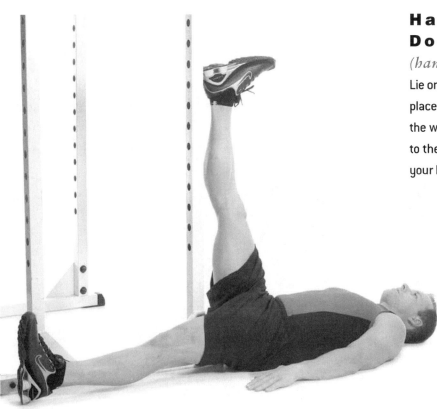

Hamstring Doorway Stretch

(hamstrings)

Lie on the floor inside a doorjamb, and place the leg closest to the door up on the wall. Try to get your hips as close to the wall as possible while keeping your legs straight.

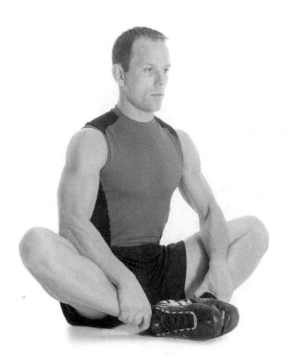

Butterfly

(adductors)

Sit with your back to a wall, and bring the soles of your feet together. With your back as straight as possible, try to bring your knees as close to the floor as you can.

Lying Hip Stretch

(glutes/piriformis)

Sit on the floor with your left leg extended and your right leg bent at 90 degrees. Next, bend your left leg back behind you, and lean your torso over your right knee as shown.

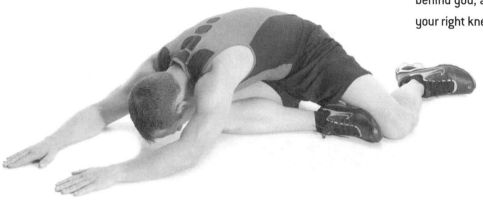

Pike Calf Stretch

(calves)

In a pike position, place the ball of your right foot on the floor, and rest the other across your right instep. Next, lower your heel, and try to get it as close to the ground as possible while keeping your right knee straight.

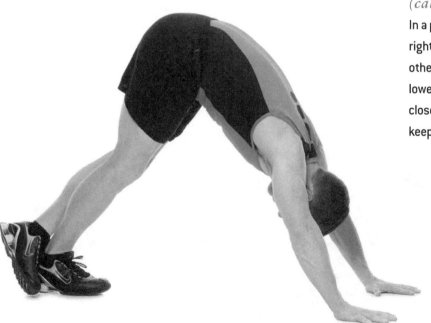

Pec Stretch

(chest)

Stand with your elbow and forearm placed on a wall or doorjamb, at or slightly below shoulder level. Then step across your body with the same side leg as the arm on the wall until you feel a stretch in your pec.

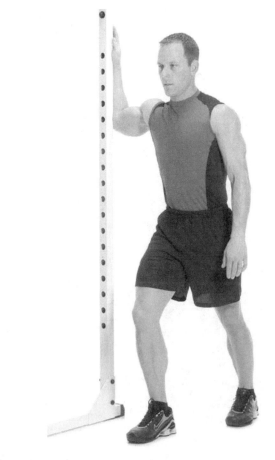

Lat Stretch

(lats)

Stand in front of a sturdy object that won't move, and grab it with both hands at about hip level. Next, bend over, and sit back into your hips until your arms are completely straight.

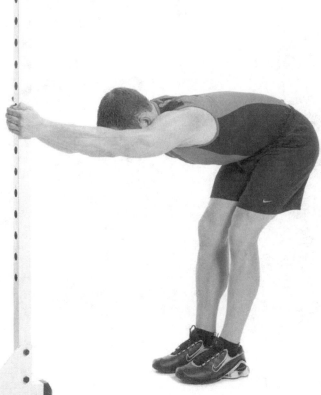

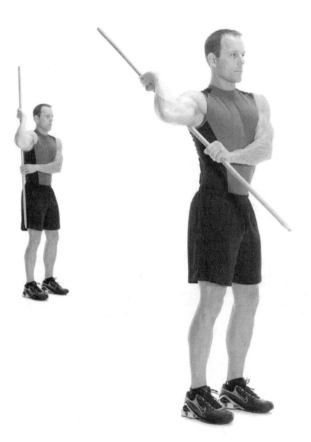

IR Broomstick Stretch

(internal rotators)

Reach over your right shoulder, and grab a broomstick as shown. Then, with your left hand, pull the bottom of the broomstick forward until you feel a stretch in your shoulder.

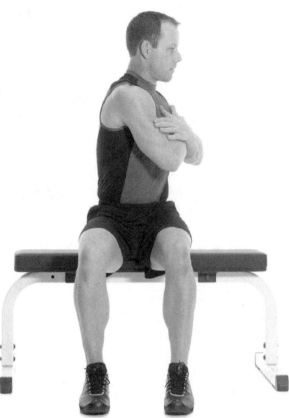

Seated Rotational Stretch

(obliques, lower back)

Sit in a chair with your legs bent 90 degrees, and turn to one side as you attempt to grab the back of the chair.

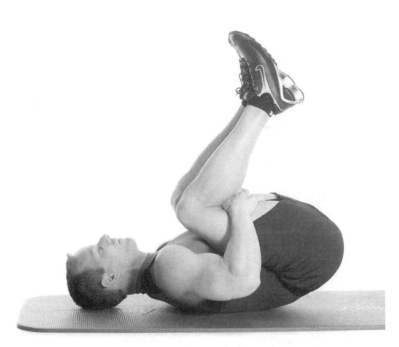

Erector Stretch
(lower back)

Lie on your back, and hug your knees into your chest as you simultaneously bring your shoulders off the ground and your head toward your knees.

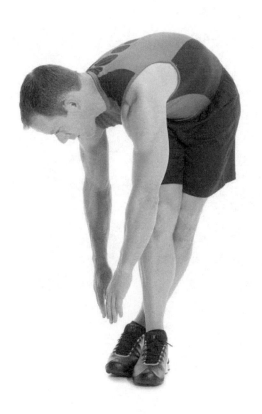

TFL/ITB Stretch
(outer thigh)

Stand with one foot crossed behind the other. Make sure the knee of the back leg is completely straight and the front knee is bent slightly. From there, lean your torso sideways away from your back leg. For example, if your left leg is back, lean to your right.

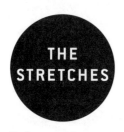

THE STRETCHES

Below we've provided you with three different mobility sequences that will help prepare you for the workouts featured in this chapter. Perform each one two or three times in circuit fashion; that is, do drills 1 to 5 in sequence before repeating them one or two more times. Although good warm-ups in their own right, they're best done after 3 to 5 minutes of large muscle group continuous activity like skipping rope or light calisthenic exercises.

Mobility Sequence #1:
>> PRIOR TO LOWER BODY WORKOUTS

1. Spidermans × 10

2. Frankensteins × 10 yards

3. Hip Walks × 10 yards

4. Gate Swings × 10 yards

5. Pike Walks × 10 yards

Mobility Sequence #2:
>> PRIOR TO UPPER BODY WORKOUTS

1. Rotational Overhead Press × 12

2. Slow Wood Chop × 12

3. Traffic Cop × 12

4. Swiss Ball Wall Rolls × 5 each arm

5. Pike Walks × 10 yards

Mobility Sequence #3:
>> PRIOR TO TOTAL BODY WORKOUTS

1. Rotational Overhead Press × 12

2. Spidermans × 10

3. Hip Walks × 10 yards

4. Slow Wood Chop × 12

5. Frankensteins × 10 yards

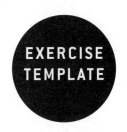
Together with all the new stretches you now know how to do, the exercises featured on this page are just what your body needs to get back into good working order. In the pages that follow, we've provided you not only with complete descriptions of how to do each properly, but we also teach you how to use this template to construct your own workouts based on *your individual needs*. If you're worried you won't know what to do, don't sweat it. It's as simple as identifying your weak points (which you've already done) and selecting the proper exercises from each column.

Lower Body Exercises

COLUMN A

》 Hip/Hamstring Dominant

Swiss Ball Leg Curls

Unilateral Deadlift

Cable Pulls Throughs

Unilateral Romanian Deadlift

COLUMN B

》 Quad Dominant

Unilateral Squat

Split Squats

COLUMN C

》 Abduction/Adduction

Plate Drags (ABD)

Plate Drags (ADD)

Low Cable (ABD)

Low Cable (ADD)

COLUMN D

》 Calves

Unilateral Calf Raises

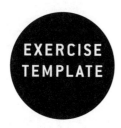

Upper Body Exercises

COLUMN E

)) Upper Back/External Rotation

Reverse Pushups

Prone Rows (elbows out)

Cable Rows (elbows out)

Reverse Flys

Cuban Presses

Side Lying External Rotation

COLUMN F

)) Chest

Bench Press with Scapular Retraction

Dips

COLUMN G

)) Core

Planks

Unanchored Situps

Russian Twists

Lateral Bridges

Swiss Ball Passes

Airplanes (lower back)

Swiss Ball Back Extensions (lower back)

The following are two different Phase I workouts based on two completely different scenarios. In the first example we use a guy with a midrange assessment score of 10 and some minor strength/ flexibility issues. Then, in the second, we concocted our own fictional physiological mess (although as some of you may soon see, this guy might not be all that fictional). Either way, you should be able to glean a lot of insight on how to construct your program based on these two examples.

Scenario #1

Assessment Score: 10 [Midrange]

Areas of concern: Knee pinching, mild internal rotation, quad dominant, flat back

Schedule: Three total-body workouts per week done on a rotating schedule, i.e., week 1: A/B/A; week 2: B/A/B

Focus: Increasing range of motion/strengthening weak links

Duration: 2 to 4 weeks

Given these parameters, you can now select from the list of exercises on page 91 according to your individual needs. For instance, your mild internal rotation of the upper arms means that you should work your upper back at either a 2:1 or 3:1 to your chest. Likewise, the fact that your knees tend to pinch inward when you squat, and you favor your quads over your hamstrings, means that you'll need to do some targeted strengthening of those hamstrings and abductors. So, in putting your workouts together, you want to pick exercises that address these concerns from the list we've provided.

Mild internal rotation: Choose 2 or 3 exercises from Column E and 1 from Column F.

Quad dominant, knee pinching: Choose 2 or 3 exercises from Column A, 1 from Column B, and 1 (ABD) from Column C.

Flat back: In addition to the deadlifts you'll already likely be doing from Column A, choose two lower-back exercises and two other exercises from Column G.

WORKOUT A

EXERCISE	SETS/REPS
Unilateral Deadlift	3 × 6–8 (each leg)*
Swiss Ball Leg Curls	2 × 6–8
Low Cable Abduction	2 × 8–10 (each leg)*
Prone Rows	3 × 8–10
Bench Press with Scapular Retraction	2 × 6–10
Airplanes	2 × 10–12
Unanchored Situps	2 × 8–10

WORKOUT B

EXERCISE	SETS/REPS
Reverse Pushups	3 × 6–8
Cuban Presses	2 × 10–12
Reverse Flys	2 × 8–10
Unilateral Romanian Deadlift	3 × 6–8 (each leg)*
Split Squats	2 × 8–10 (each leg)*
Swiss Ball Back Extensions	2 × 8–10
Planks	2 × 20–30 seconds

Whether or not you do the same number of sets on each leg depends upon whether or not there is an imbalance from one side to the other. If an imbalance exists, do at least one more set for the weaker side.

STRETCHES TO BE DONE AT LEAST 3 OR 4 TIMES PER WEEK

MILD INTERNAL ROTATION: Doorway Pec Stretch, IR Broomstick Stretch

KNEE PINCHING: Butterfly (Adductors), TFL/ITB Stretch

FLAT BACK: Hamstring Doorway Stretch

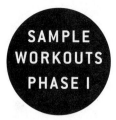

Scenario #2

Assessment Score: 14 [High]

Areas of concentration: Heavy internal rotation, tight hip flexors, knees bowing, weak core/limited rotation. Three workouts per week done on a rotating schedule, i.e., upper/lower/upper; lower/upper/lower

Focus: Same as on page 93.

Duration: 4 weeks +

Heavy internal rotation: Choose 3 or 4 exercises from Column E and none from Column F.

Tight hip flexors/knee bowing: Choose 2 or 3 exercises from Column A, 1 from Column C, and only 1 from Column B, which will be done only once every other week.

Core/limited rotation: Choose 4 or 5 exercises from Column G.

LOWER BODY

EXERCISE	SETS/REPS
Unilateral Romanian Deadlift	3 × 6–8 (each leg)*
Swiss Ball Leg Curls	2–3 × 6–8
Plate Drags (Add)	2 × 10–12 (each leg)*
Unilateral Squat	2 × 6–8 (each leg)**
Unilateral Calf Raises	2 × 8–10 (each leg)
Unanchored Situps	2 × 8–10
Planks	3 × 20–30 seconds

UPPER BODY

EXERCISE	SETS/REPS
Reverse Pushups	3 × 6–8
Cable Rows	3 × 8–10
Reverse Flys	2 × 10–12
Side Lying External Rotation	2 × 10–12*
Swiss Ball Passes	2 × 6–8
Russian Twists	2 × 4–6 (each side)
Lateral Bridges	2 × 8–10 (each side)

Whether or not you do the same number of sets on each leg depends upon whether or not there is an imbalance from one side to the other. If an imbalance exists, do at least one more set for the weaker side.

** *To be done every other week*

STRETCHES TO BE DONE ON A DAILY BASIS

HEAVY INTERNAL ROTATION: Doorway Pec Stretch, IR Broomstick Stretch

TIGHT HIP FLEXORS/KNEE BOWING: Three Point Stretch, Lying Hip Stretch

WEAK CORE/LIMITED ROTATION: Seated Rotational Stretch

»Lower Body

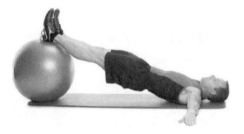

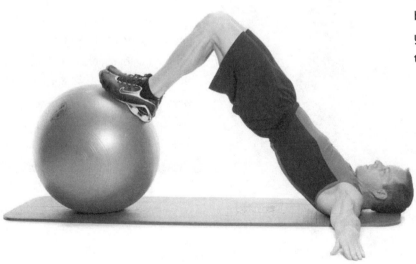

Swiss Ball Leg Curls

(hamstrings, glutes)

Lie on your back with your heels and lower calves on a Swiss Ball. First lift your hips up until your body forms a ramp; then pull the ball in toward you by bending your knees and extending your hips. Pause for a second, and then slowly reverse the sequence.

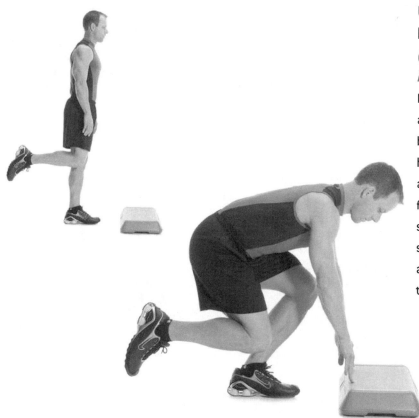

Unilateral Deadlift

(glutes, hamstrings, erectors)

From a standing position, bend one leg at a 90-degree angle, and hold it up behind you. Begin by dropping your hips back and then bending your knee as you lower your hips toward the floor. Your back can round slightly, since you're not under load. Once the shin grazes the floor (or you've gotten as low as you can), press back up to the starting position.

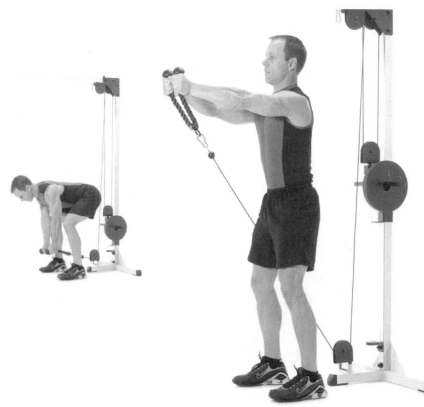

Cable Pull Throughs

(hamstrings, glutes, erectors)

Stand with your back to a cable station, approximately 1 to 2 feet in front of it. Reach between your legs, and grab the handle by bending your knees and keeping your back fairly straight. To get the weight up, drive your feet into the ground, and bring your hips forward as you straighten your torso. In the top position, your arms should be no higher than parallel to the ground. Pause, and slowly lower the weight back to the starting position.

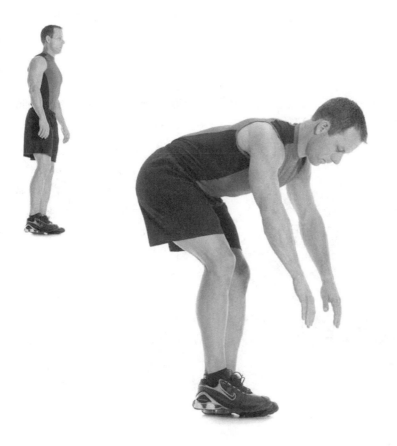

Unilateral Romanian Deadlift

(hamstrings, glutes, erectors)

From a standing position, lift one foot an inch or two off the ground, while maintaining a slight bend in the support knee. Next, drive your hips back as you begin to lean forward until your torso is as close to parallel to the floor as possible. Be sure your support knee doesn't bend any more or your back round as you lower yourself forward. Keep a slight bend in the knee and a slight arch in your lower back.

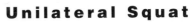

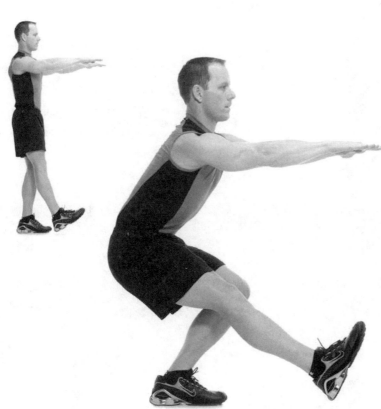

Unilateral Squat

(quads, hamstrings, erectors)

From a standing position, raise one leg off the floor, and hold it out in front of you approximately 6 to 12 inches off the floor. Next, allow your arms to come forward, as you bend your supporting knee and hip and lower yourself down as low as possible. Once there, pause, and press back up, making sure to hold the other leg out in front of you the entire time.

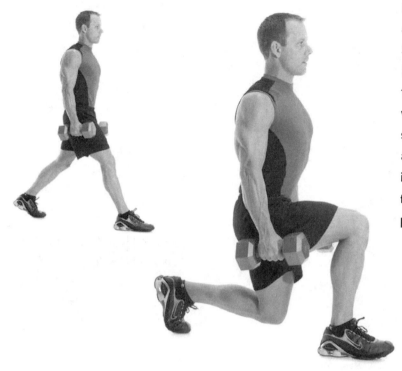

Split Squats

(quads, hamstrings, and glutes)

Stand with one leg approximately 3 to 3½ feet in front of the other, with only the ball of your back foot in contact with the floor. Keeping your torso as straight as possible, bend both knees, and descend toward the floor so that in the bottom position, your lead leg forms a 90-degree angle. Pause, and press back up to the starting position.

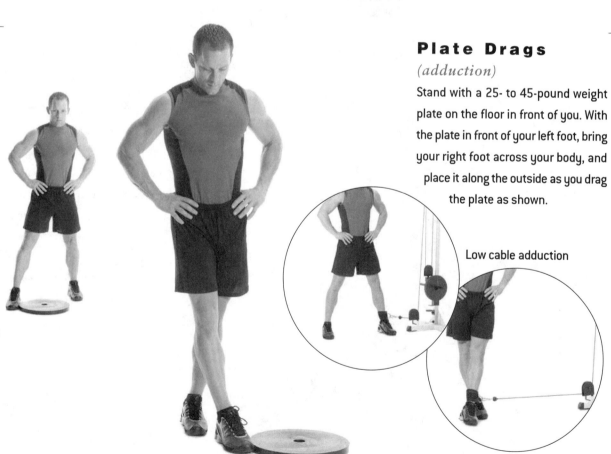

Plate Drags

(adduction)

Stand with a 25- to 45-pound weight plate on the floor in front of you. With the plate in front of your left foot, bring your right foot across your body, and place it along the outside as you drag the plate as shown.

Low cable adduction

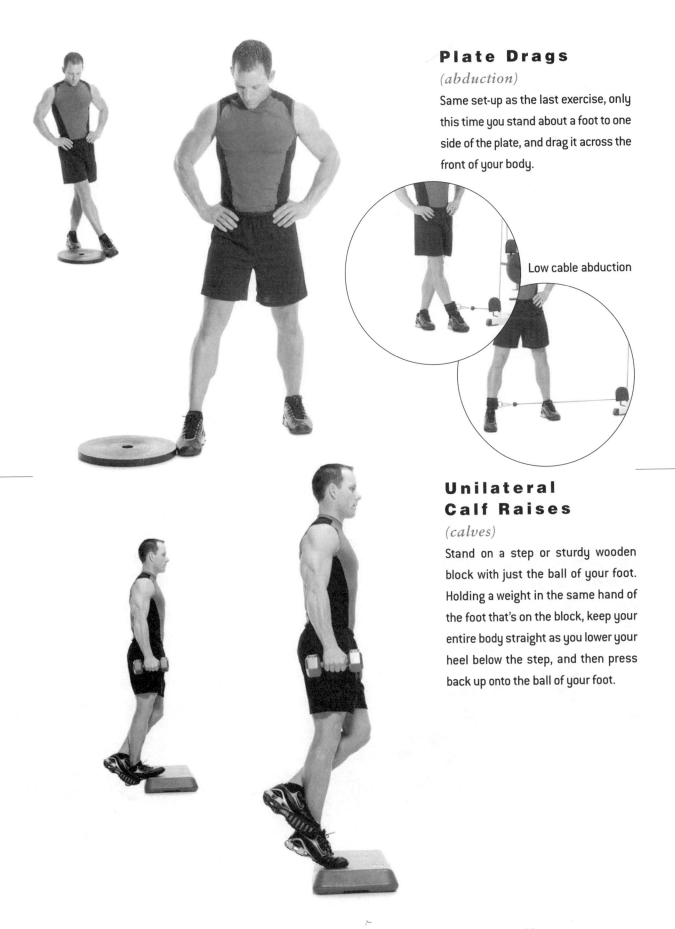

Plate Drags

(abduction)

Same set-up as the last exercise, only this time you stand about a foot to one side of the plate, and drag it across the front of your body.

Low cable abduction

Unilateral Calf Raises

(calves)

Stand on a step or sturdy wooden block with just the ball of your foot. Holding a weight in the same hand of the foot that's on the block, keep your entire body straight as you lower your heel below the step, and then press back up onto the ball of your foot.

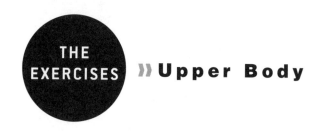

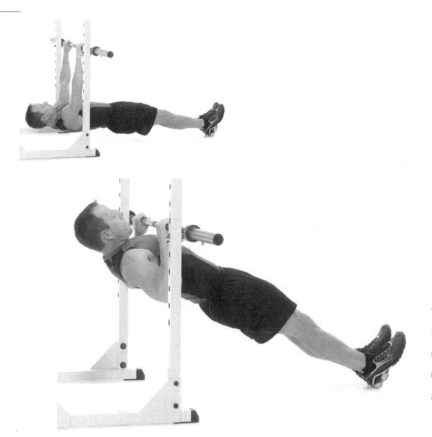

Reverse Pushups
(upper back, biceps)

Lie underneath a barbell set in the supports in the squat rack (how high the bar is depends on how strong you are; the higher up you place it, the easier the exercise is to do). Grasp the bar with a false grip (thumbs around the bar with the rest of the fingers), and support your weight on the backs of your heels as shown. Next, lift your hips so your body forms a straight line, and with your elbows held out to the sides, pull yourself up toward the bar. At the top, your chest should be as close to the bar as possible. Lower yourself until your arms are straight, and repeat.

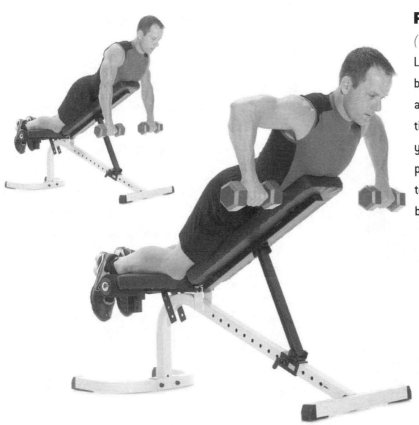

Prone Rows
(upper back, biceps)

Lie prone over a 45-degree incline bench holding a couple of dumbbells at arm's length. With your palms positioned so they face behind you, pinch your shoulder blades together, and pull the weights up to the sides of your torso. Hold for a second, and lower back to the starting position.

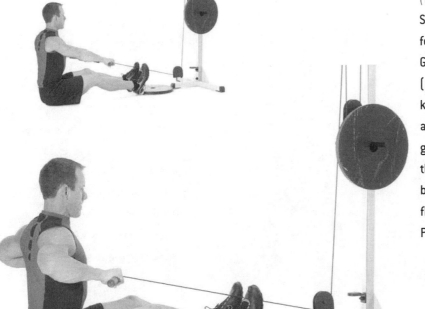

Cable Rows
(upper back, biceps)

Sit in front of a cable station with your feet up against the support plate. Grabbing the bar with a pronated (palms facing away from you) grip, keep your torso right over your hips, and pinch your shoulder blades together as you pull the bar in toward the base of your sternum (breast bone). Be sure to keep your elbows flared out, away from your body. Pause for a second, and repeat.

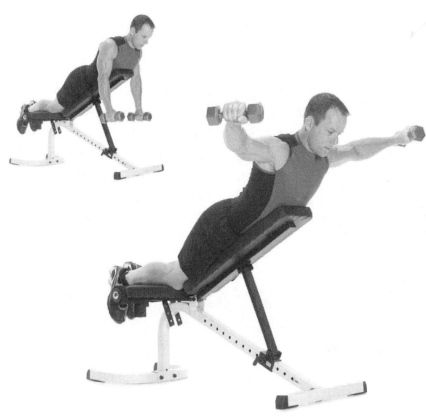

Reverse Flys

(rear deltoids, upper back)

Lie prone over a 45-degree exercise bench holding a pair of dumbbells at arm's length. Keeping a slight bend in your elbows, pinch your shoulder blades together, and work your arms up in a wide, arcing motion. At the top of the movement, your elbows should remain slightly bent, and you should see the weights out of the corner of your eyes.

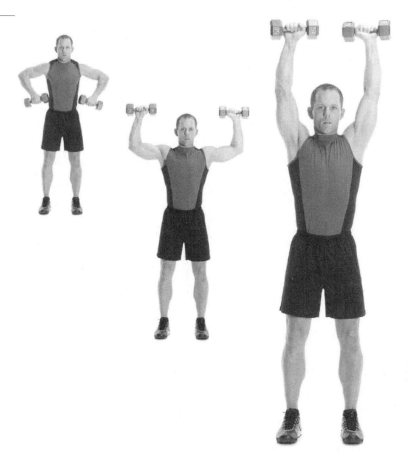

Cuban Presses

(external rotators, shoulders, triceps)

Stand holding a pair of light dumbbells with your arms bent about 90 degrees and out in line with your shoulders. Beginning with your forearms pointing down toward the ground, keep your upper arms still, and rotate the weights up until your forearms are pointed toward the ceiling. From there, press the dumbbells straight up overhead before lowering them back down and repeating the sequence.

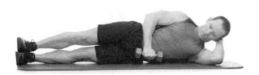

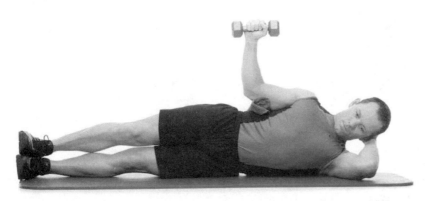

Side Lying External Rotation

(external rotators)

Lie on the floor on one side with your elbow bent 90 degrees. Holding a light dumbbell in your hand, rotate your forearm until your arm is as close to perpendicular to the ground as you can get it. Be sure to maintain a neutral wrist, and avoid cocking your hand back in an attempt to increase your range of motion. Placing a rolled-up towel between your elbow and hip can help maintain proper shoulder angle.

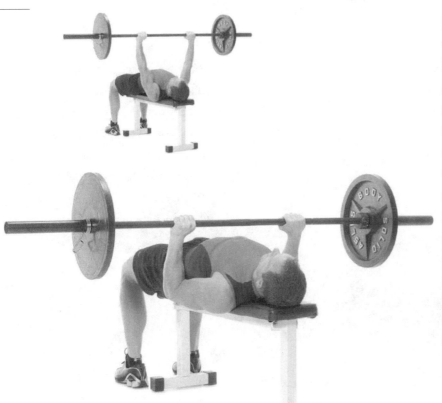

Bench Press with Scapular Retraction

(chest, shoulders, triceps, upper back)

Lie on a bench as if you're about to execute a set of flat presses. Next, grasp the bar, but before you begin, pinch your shoulder blades together on the bench. Maintain this position throughout the entire exercise, even when pressing the bar up. Begin by unracking the bar and lowering it down to the appropriate depth (see page 33). Pause for a second before pressing the weight back up.

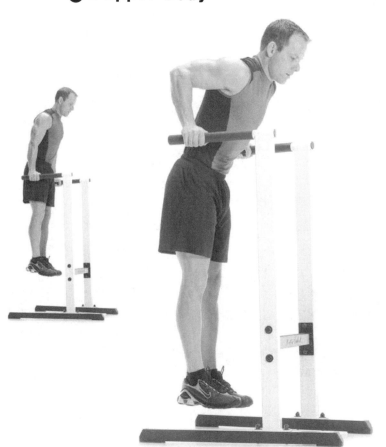

Dips
(chest, shoulders, triceps)

Prop yourself up at arm's length on a set of parallel dipping bars. Begin by lowering yourself down toward the floor to a point where your upper arms are parallel to the bars. Pause for a second, and press back up.

✓ Planks
(TVA)

Assume a pushup position, but instead of having your arms straight, rest your weight on your forearms. Next, suck in your belly button, and contract your glutes to flatten the arch in your lower back. Now hold this position for 20 to 30 seconds without allowing your back to arch.

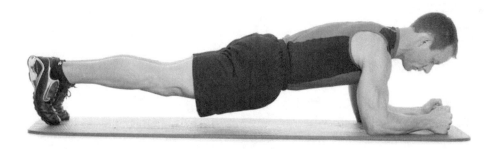

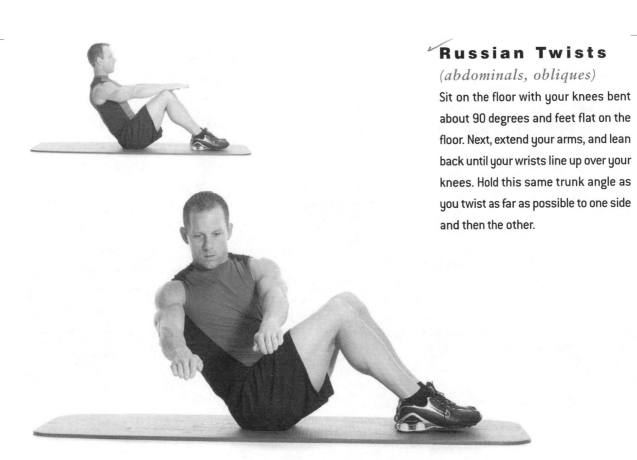

Unanchored Situps

(abdominals, hip flexors)

Lie on the floor with your knees bent about 90 degrees and your feet flat. Keeping your arms at your sides or folded across your chest, use your abdominals to pull yourself up to a seated position. Hold for a second, and lower back down under control.

Russian Twists

(abdominals, obliques)

Sit on the floor with your knees bent about 90 degrees and feet flat on the floor. Next, extend your arms, and lean back until your wrists line up over your knees. Hold this same trunk angle as you twist as far as possible to one side and then the other.

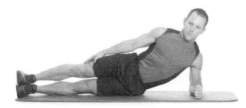

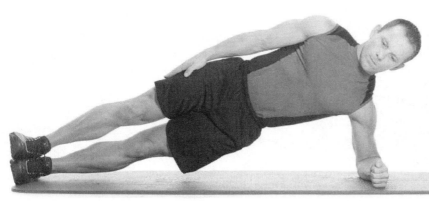

Lateral Bridges
(obliques, abdominals)

Lie on your side with your forearm lined upright beneath your shoulder, perpendicular to your torso. Keeping your body totally straight, contract your abdominals and obliques as you raise your lower torso, hips, and legs off the floor. In the top position, your body should form a diagonal line from your feet to your head.

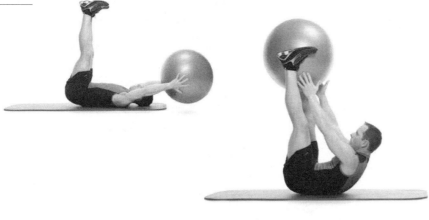

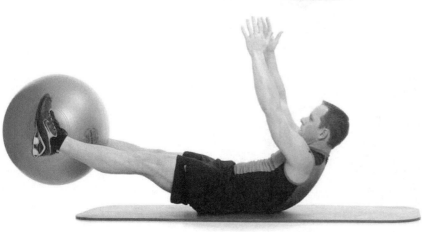

Swiss Ball Passes
(abdominals, hip flexors)

Lie on the floor with your arms outstretched behind you holding a Swiss Ball. With your legs held straight up over your hips, lift your torso off the floor, and place the ball between your feet. Next, keeping your torso off the ground and your arms extended, lower your legs as far toward the floor as you can without allowing your lower back to arch. Once you reach this point, use your abdominals and hip flexors to bring the ball back up to your hands, and then lower yourself back to the starting position.

Airplanes

(lower and upper back, glutes, and hamstrings)

Lie facedown on the floor with your legs straight and your arms outstretched in line with your shoulders. Begin by simultaneously lifting your legs and upper torso off the ground. As you do, pinch your shoulder blades together to activate your upper back.

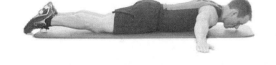

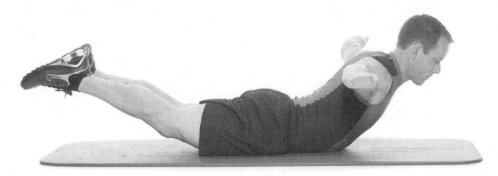

Swiss Ball Back Extensions

(lower back)

Lie prone over a Swiss Ball with your legs straight and your torso rounded over the surface of the ball. With your hands folded behind your back, use your spinal erectors to extend your spine and lift your chest completely off the ball.

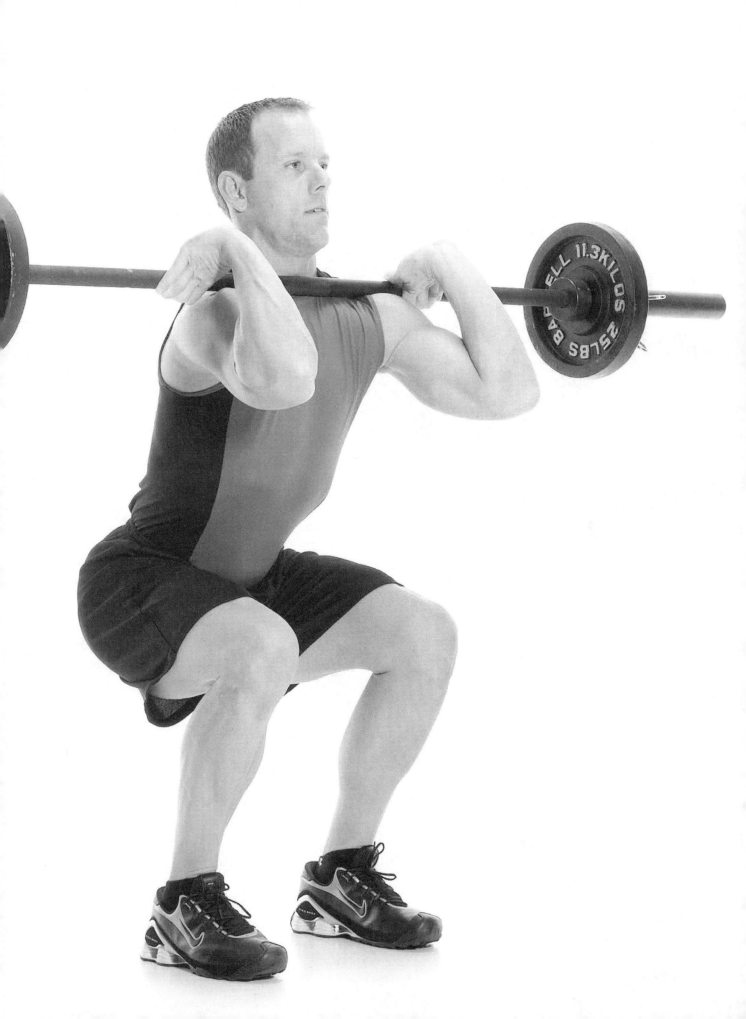

TRAINING: PHASE II

After the previous corrective/preparatory phase, your body should be feeling and moving noticeably better than it ever has before. Take that last phase seriously, and you'll be more flexible, stronger in all the right places, and best of all, finally ready to get down to the business of building some serious muscle. That's right, the goal of this phase is to increase muscle hypertrophy, albeit not in the traditional manner. Noticeably absent are the biceps curls and leg extensions that clutter other programs; the exercises featured in this chapter are far more inclusive than that. By forcing you to recruit large amounts of muscle mass, they not only give you more "bang for your buck," but they also help set the stage for the more intensive strength work to follow in Phase III. We do this by design, with each phase building on the one before it, leading up to the ultimate muscle-building crescendo in Phase IV.

Besides the exercises themselves, the other thing that's different about our hypertrophy phase compared with others is the loading protocol. As some of you who've been training for a while may have heard, working with weights in the 8- to 12-repetition range is supposed to provide the "optimal" muscle-building stimulus. Our question is, optimal for whom? Certainly not you muscularly challenged types, that's for sure. Once you can lift a weight for that number of reps, you're creating a far less potent stimulus for your type IIb muscle fibers; remember them? If you're looking to bulk up, these hypertrophy-prone guys need to be your primary area of focus. And the best way to get these fibers growing is with heavy weights and relatively low reps.

Enter the classic 5 × 5 lifting regimen. As you may have guessed, it calls for you to do five sets of five reps for each exercise. If you're wondering whether this would add up to far too much volume for a guy who has a tough time building muscle, let us describe the rest of the workout. You're actually only going to be employing this set and rep scheme with two major lifts each time you train. The rest of your workout will be comprised of a couple of sets of assistance exercises to help ensure more balanced development. The premise here is simple: Keep loading high, volume low to moderate, and target the muscle fibers with the greatest potential for growth.

There are just a few things we'd like to mention before you get started:

》 Exercise selection: The exercises in this phase were selected because they work, plain and simple. Try to stick with them as best you can. If you can't do one or two due to equipment limitations, feel free to substitute with a similar exercise (i.e., if your gym doesn't have a squat rack, choose a new gym, but in the meantime, the leg press will work). If you can't do an exercise because of a chronic injury (i.e., you can't do dips because of a shoulder impingement), we suggest you either extend the duration of your corrective phase, or consider physical rehabilitation to correct the problem. If you simply won't do an exercise because you "hate it," that's not a valid excuse, so do it anyway.

》 Loading: Here's how 5×5 works: Select a weight that allows you to get no more than five or, at the very most, six reps. Between sets, rest for 2 to 2½ minutes. Repeat the same load again until the five sets have been completed. If you can't get all five reps for each set, just do what you can. When you can eventually get all five sets with a given weight, increase it by 5 percent on your next workout, and continue to do so every time you complete all 25 reps. For the assistance exercises, because many involve a postural component, it's all right to increase the rep range slightly (6 to 8 per set) to tap into some of your more endurance-based fibers.

》 Rest intervals: As we just mentioned, 2 minutes should suffice between each set in the 5×5 protocol. For all other exercises, limit your rest to 90 seconds between sets. If you're the type who recovers quickly between sets and is looking for a way to increase the intensity slightly, instead of doing them as straight sets, try supersetting your 5×5 exercises. So, for example, you might do a five-rep front squat, rest 60 to 90 seconds, and go into a five-rep incline bench press. Then, rest 60 to 90 seconds; go back to the front squat and so on until all 10 sets are complete. The cool part is even though you only rested say, 90 seconds after the squat, you're still resting your lower body in the time it takes you to get to the bench, set up, do your set, get back to squat rack, and rest another 60 to 90 seconds. When it's all said and done, you will have rested a full 3½ minutes before you attempt that front squat again. Keep in mind, though, that this is for advanced trainees only because your central nervous system is still being stressed, despite the fact you're working different segments of your body.

》 Supplemental activity: Seeing as how your primary goal in this phase is to build muscle, you've got to be somewhat Spartan in your extracurricular activities. Try to limit outside sport activities. For your cardiovascular/aerobic work, you should be doing two additional 12- to 15-minute cardiovascular workouts. Keep the intensity high to increase the cardiovascular stimulus and the duration short so as not to burn too much energy (see Chapter 5 for the specific workouts to complement this phase).

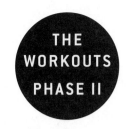

The exercises in this section are divided into three separate workouts (A, B, and C), which are best done in order with at least one day of rest in between them. So, a typical week might look like Workout A on Monday, Workout B on Wednesday, and Workout C on Friday. It is permissible to occasionally take two full days off between workouts; just make sure you get in all three each week.

WORKOUT A

EXERCISE	SETS/REPS
Barbell Front Squat	5 × 5
Incline Bench Press	5 × 5
Bulgarian Split Squat	2 × 6–8
One Arm Row (elbow out)	2 × 6–8

WORKOUT B

EXERCISE	SETS/REPS
Chinup*	5 × 5
Hang Clean & Press	5 × 5
Cable Pull Throughs	2 × 6–8
Weighted Situps	2 × 6–8

WORKOUT C

EXERCISE	SETS/REPS
Elevated Trap Bar D-Lift	5 × 5
Dips	5 × 5
Cable Rows	2 × 6–8
Reverse Hypers	2 × 6–8

Add weight if necessary.

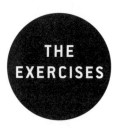
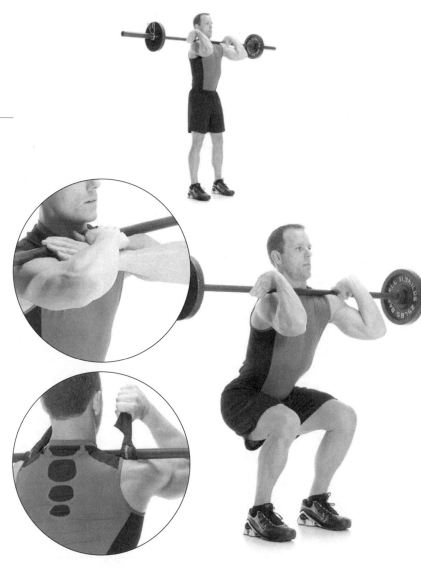

Barbell Front Squat

(quads, hamstrings, spinal erectors)

Walk into a squat rack with a barbell set at about collarbone level. Rest the bar on the front deltoids with the bar lightly touching your throat. You have three different options: Cross your arms, and place each hand over the opposite shoulder. Use a clean grip or place a pair of lifting straps around the bar, and hold them up. Once you've supported the bar, walk back a few steps and set your feet slightly wider than shoulder width apart. Break at the knee first, then the hips, and maintain an arch in your lower back. Descend as low as you can while still maintaining a slight arch and an upright torso. Pause for a second, and return the weight to the starting position.

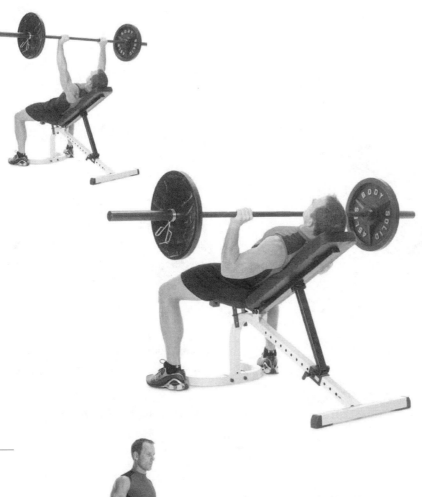

Close Grip Incline Bench Press

(chest, front deltoids, triceps)

Lie on an incline bench, and grasp the bar with a close (14- to 18-inch) grip. With your feet flat on the floor, lift the bar off the supports, and lower it toward your upper chest. Once you've reached the appropriate depth, pause for a second, and press the bar back up.

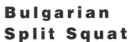

Bulgarian Split Squat

(quads, hamstrings, glutes)

Stand with your back to an exercise bench running perpendicular to your body. Reach back, and place the instep of your back foot on the bench, as you support your weight on your front foot. Keeping your torso as straight as possible, bend both knees until your front leg forms a 90-degree angle. Pause, and press back up.

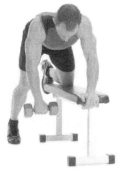

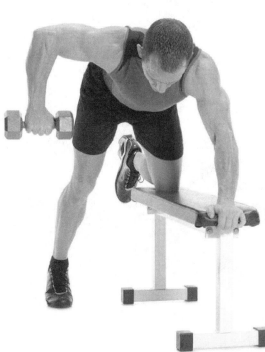

One Arm Row, elbow out

(upper back, biceps)

Support yourself on an exercise bench by placing your knee and hand of the same side on the bench and the other leg on the floor. Make sure your back is flat like a three-legged table. Next, with your free hand, grasp a dumbbell with a false grip, and let it hang at arm's length beneath your shoulder with your palm facing behind you. Begin by drawing your elbow up past your torso by pinching your shoulder blade in toward your spine. Avoid twisting or contorting your body to get the weight up.

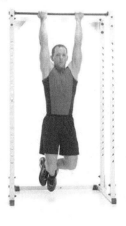

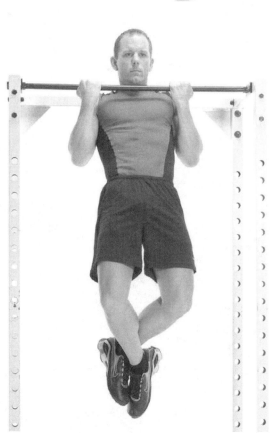

Chinup

(upper back, biceps)

Grasp an overhead bar with a false grip and your hands approximately shoulder width apart. From a dead hang, stick your chest out, and pull yourself up to the bar until your chin clears the bar (or your chest touches, if you have the strength). Lower, and repeat.

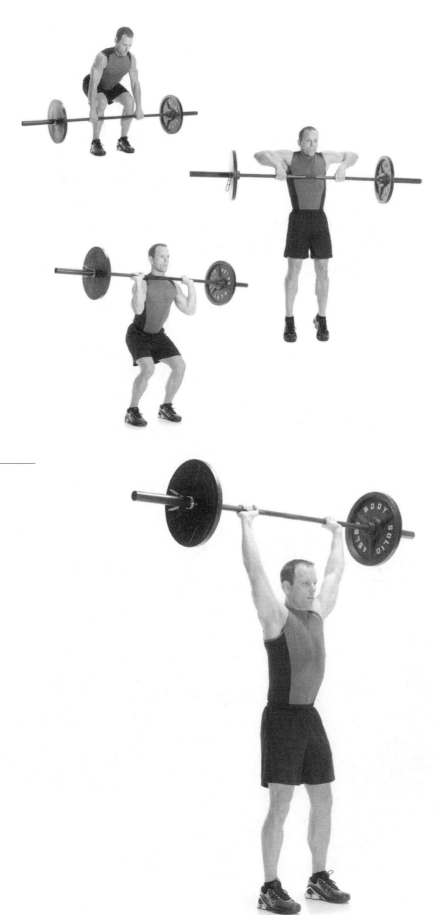

Hang Clean & Press
(upper back, trapezius, biceps, shoulders, triceps)

Stand holding a barbell at arm's length in front of you. With your knees bent and your back arched so that the bar starts off just above knee level, quickly extend your hips, knees, and ankles as you simultaneously shrug your shoulders up as high as you can. Continue this wave of power by quickly pulling the bar up the front of your body toward your chin. Once the bar clears your chest, immediately "drop" under it, and catch it across your front deltoids in a front squat position. You then extend your knees, and press the bar overhead in one continuous motion. Lower the bar back to the shoulders, flip it down, and repeat.

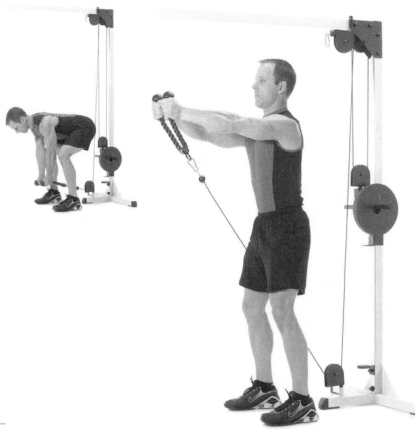

Cable Pull Throughs

(hamstrings, glutes, erectors)

Stand with your back to a cable station approximately 1 to 2 feet in front of it. Reach between your legs, and grab the handle by bending your knees and keeping your back fairly straight. To get the weight up, drive your feet into the ground, and bring your hips forward as you straighten your torso. In the top position, your arms should be no higher than parallel to the ground. Pause, and slowly lower the weight back to the starting position.

Weighted Situps

(abdominal wall, hip flexors, and lower back)

Lie down on the floor with your knees bent and your feet flat. Holding a weight across your chest, sit up until your forearms touch your thighs using as little momentum as possible. Pause for a second, and repeat. *Note:* This exercise can be done with or without the feet anchored underneath something for support, with the latter being much more difficult.

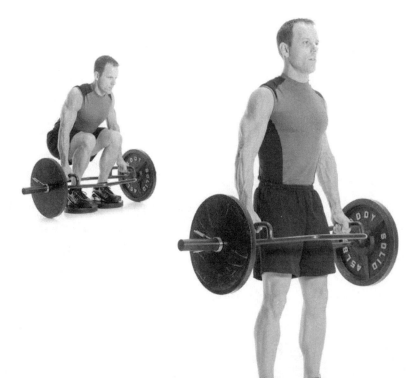

Elevated Trap Bar Deadlift

(glutes, hamstrings, quads, upper back, lower back)

Note: How high you elevate your feet depends on your flexibility and the length of your limbs. Some of you may use a 4-inch block, while others may only be able to use a pair of 25-pound plates. The objective of elevating the feet is to increase glute and hamstring involvement. Standing on whichever device you choose, grasp the bar with a full grip, and keep your torso as erect as possible. Next, drive the bar up by pushing your feet through the floor and extending your hips forward. Once in the standing position, lower the weight back down to the floor, and repeat.

Dips

(chest, shoulders, triceps)

Prop yourself up at arm's length on a set of parallel dipping bars. Begin by lowering yourself down toward the floor to a point where your upper arms are parallel to the bars. Pause for a second, and press back up.

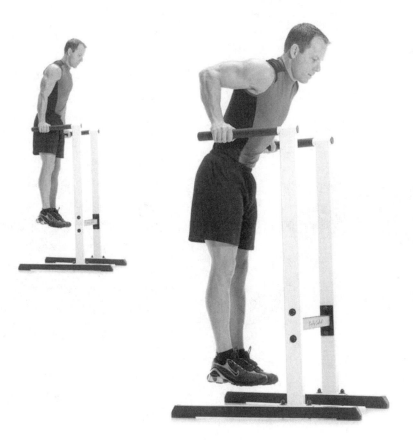

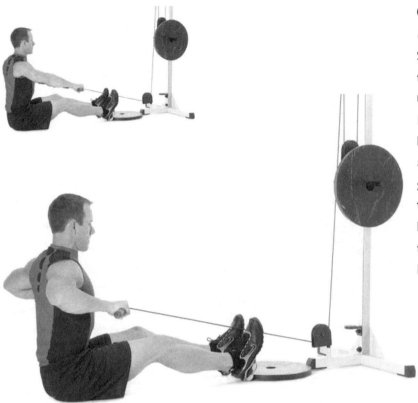

Cable Rows
(upper back, biceps)

Sit in front of a cable station with your feet up against the support plate. Grabbing the bar with a pronated (palms facing away from you) grip, keep your torso right over your hips, and pinch your shoulder blades together as you pull the bar in toward the base of your sternum (breast bone). Be sure to keep your elbows flared out, away from your body. Pause for a second, and repeat.

Reverse Hypers
(glutes, hamstrings, spinal erectors)

Use a Roman chair, and position yourself opposite from the way you would if you were doing a back extension (i.e., hips on the pad, legs hanging off, and arms outstretched to grab onto the supports). Keeping your legs perfectly straight, raise them until they're parallel to (or slightly higher than) the floor. Pause for a second, and lower them back down until they're just short of perpendicular to the floor. *Note:* Loading can be tough here. If you're able to use more than body weight, and you don't have access to the specific machine, use ankle weights or have someone place a medicine ball or light dumbbell between your feet.

Think of it this way, your instincts haven't exactly proven right up to this point. Don't feel bad though—you're not alone. Most scrawny guys we've encountered in weight rooms far and wide almost always make the mistake of thinking that doing more work is better. Maybe it's because their bodies are better suited to endurance-based tasks, but for some strange reason, they seem hell-bent on testing the limits of what they can physically withstand. That's great when you're training for a marathon or triathlon, but it's not the way to go about becoming bigger and stronger. So, please, as much as you think you know what your body needs, resist the urge to do more and put your faith in us.

This workout is simple and intense. Yet, while simple, it contains everything you need to start packing on some size. There's no need to add to it or do it more frequently than the number of times it's been prescribed. In fact, not only isn't there a need, you're a fool if you do add to it. Remember, in some instances, more isn't necessarily better. For a guy like you, training is usually one of those instances.

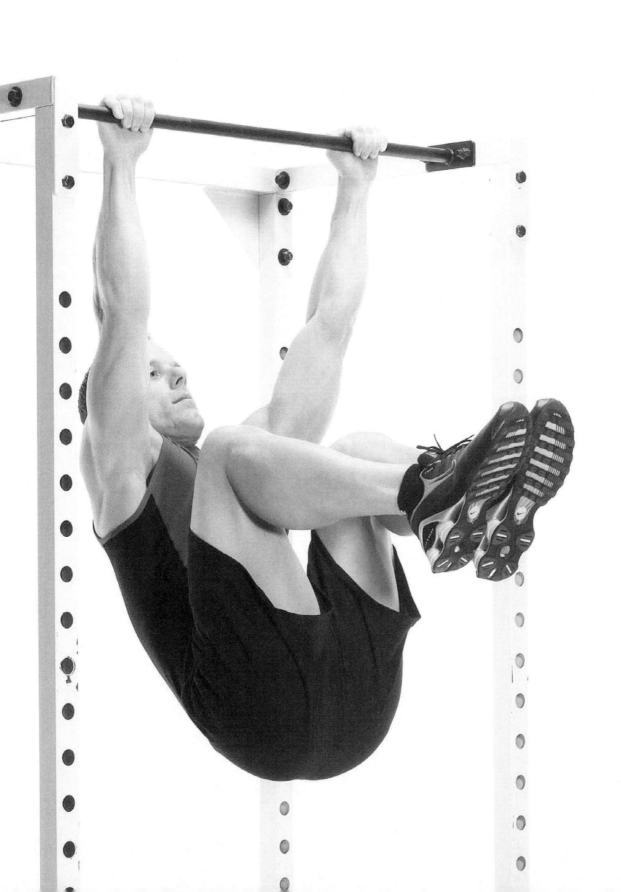

TRAINING: PHASE III

If you thought you were handling some heavy loads in the previous phase, better brace yourself. For the next 4 weeks, you're going to be pushing weights that are pretty near maximal. For many of you, this will be a completely new experience. That's because the majority of guys who train with weights care more about the way they look than how much they can lift. That's too bad because increasing strength is one of the easiest ways to get bigger. How's that, you ask? Well, when you increase your maximal strength, you also end up increasing your submaximal strength as a byproduct. This means you'll be able to lift more weight for a given number of reps, and the more weight you can lift, the greater the stimulus for growth. Here's how it works.

Let's say your 1 repetition maximum (1RM) on the bench press is 200 pounds. Now, if your goal is to increase muscle mass, you're obviously going to be working with a weight that allows you to perform more than one repetition. Sure, lower repetitions (one to three) are great for improving nervous system function, and they really recruit those all-important type IIb muscle fibers. Trouble is, your overall training volume would be too low. To build muscle, you'd be better off selecting a weight somewhere in the neighborhood of 80 to 85 percent of this amount (or in this case, 160 to 170 pounds) to allow for a slightly higher rep range (four to eight) and greater overall training volume.

Now let's say that after completing an intensive strength phase like the one featured in this chapter, you get your 1RM up to 220 pounds. Assuming that you'll once again work in that 80 to 85 percent range, that means you'll now be handling 176 to 187 pounds *for the same number of reps*. Hmm, do you suppose that loading your muscles with 16 to 17 more pounds over what essentially equates to the same time frame might lead to superior growth? Bottom line: You want to get bigger? Get stronger!

RIDE THE WAVE

Making the case for including a strength phase in what is essentially a bodybuilding program is the easy part. The hard part is trying to determine the most efficient loading protocol to use. Remember, we're only talking 4 weeks here, so we need something that will deliver maximum results in minimal time. That's why we decided to go with the one system that practically guarantees substantial improvements in strength by basically tricking your nervous system into working more efficiently. It's called wave loading, and it is, without question, one of the most effective and interesting strength protocols out there.

Although there are a number of different ways to do it, the variation we've selected requires you to divide each of your major lifts into two, or more, separate "waves," comprised of three sets of descending reps. So, for example, in Wave 1, you'll do four reps in the first set, three in the second, and two in the third. The key being that you don't go all out on any of these sets. You'll take care of that in Wave 2, where you'll once again do four, three, and two reps, only this time with more weight than the first go-round. Although some opt to include a third, or possibly even a fourth wave, we feel it wise to limit you to two, especially considering that you'll be using this protocol with two major lifts per workout. Due to the long rest intervals and heavy nervous system demand, we're confident this is the best way to go. Here's an example of what a typical wave progression might look like using the squat.

Current 2 rep max = 300 pounds

Wave 1

4 × 275/rest 3 minutes

3 × 285/rest 3 minutes

2 × 295/rest 3 minutes

Wave 2

4 × 285/rest 3 minutes

3 × 295/rest 3 minutes

2 × 305

As you can see, in just one workout, you can potentially surpass your previous 2RM. Notice that we say potentially; that's because in order for you to reap the full benefit of this program, there are a few things you have to make sure you do. First and foremost is that you need to establish what your 1RM is for each of the lifts in this program (see "What's Your Type?" on page 50). Granted, for some of you, this will be a rather daunting task. We mentioned in the beginning of this chapter that a lot of guys don't train for strength. Assuming you're one of them, trying to figure out the maximal amount of weight you can lift can be about as much fun as a trip to the dentist on tax day. It is, however, integral to your ability to follow through with this program, so do your best to come up with as accurate an assessment as possible. Just be sure you're intimately familiar with the form for each lift before attempting to do so.

There are only two other things that can sabotage your progress while on this program. One of them is going too heavy on the first wave. The reason that wave loading is so effective for increasing strength is that the first wave serves to disinhibit your nervous system, which, in turn, acts as sort of a primer for subsequent waves. It's kind of like the way having a few drinks at the annual Christmas party lowers your social inhibitions. Only this time, instead of making regrettable comments to coworkers, you end up lifting more weight than you have previously. Because your nervous system is so jacked up from the first wave, by the time the second one rolls around, it's ready for the main event. That is, provided, of course, you didn't push too hard on the first wave, at which point all bets are off. If this is the case, you'll be lucky to even replicate the same poundage on wave two. This is one of the main reasons you need to get your 1RM numbers right.

So exactly how do you go about selecting the right weight so you don't push too hard on the first wave? If you have a little experience working with heavy loads, starting off with as much as 85 to 90 percent of your 1RM and adding weight at each set would be fine for the first wave, being sure of course to up the weight accordingly for wave two. On the other hand, those of you for whom this may be new ground will probably want to be less aggressive initially, using say 80 percent or so on the first wave and upping the weight slightly from there. Keep in mind, it's not an exact science; just be sure that the weight continues to climb and you're working with weights beyond your previous 1RM for multiple reps by the end of the program.

The other surefire way to screw up your results is failing to take enough rest between sets. We realize those long rest intervals between sets might have you feeling a little bit uneasy. In fact, we can almost hear you saying things like "Wow, 3 minutes between sets? Isn't that too much?" Keep in mind, this isn't circuit training or cardio. You're trying to build strength here, not stay in your target heart rate zone. Since your central nervous system

takes longer to restore between sets than your muscles do, you'll need every minute to improve upon your first wave. So even if you feel you can lift again after just a minute or two, don't! As for what to do with all that downtime between sets, try some positive visualization or maybe some low-intensity dynamic flexibility drills to stay limber. Whatever you do, though, try to stay "in the zone." When you're training for strength, you need total focus and concentration. So don't use your rest periods to chat about last night's game or keep up with the latest stock quotes.

Finally, although the overall work volume will be somewhat low during this phase, the energy demand on the nervous system is high. In other words, don't expect to do a whole lot more once you've completed your two major lifts. A few light sets of some basic assistance exercises will be all you need to round out your training sessions. Doing more would be a mistake, as it would extend your training time and likely compromise your recuperative powers to some degree. So do us a favor, and just stick to the program. As with the previous phase, a couple of brief, intense cardio workouts are permissible on off days from training. Just make sure they're as far removed from your workouts as possible, i.e., try to avoid a cardio session the morning after an evening strength workout.

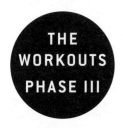

The exercises in this section are also divided into three separate workouts (A, B, and C), however, unlike the protocol from Phase II, you may find that the heavier loads and increased nervous system demand make it necessary to take two full days off between each workout. So, a sample week might look like Workout A on Monday, Workout B on Thursday, and Workout C on Sunday, with Workout A not being repeated again until the following Wednesday. You then simply continue with this cycle.

WORKOUT A

EXERCISE	SETS/REPS
Trap Bar Deadlift	2 × 4/3/2
Flat Bench Press	2 × 4/3/2
Cable External Rotation	2 × 10–12
Barbell Rollouts	2 × 8–10

WORKOUT B

EXERCISE	SETS/REPS
Hang Snatch	2 × 4/3/2
Military Press	2 × 4/3/2
Russian Twists	2 × 8–10
Prone Row	2 × 8–10

WORKOUT C

EXERCISE	SETS/REPS
Box Squat	2 × 4/3/2
Pullups*	2 × 4/3/2
Hanging Leg Raises	2 × 8–10
Cable Rows to Neck	2 × 8–10

Add weight if necessary.

Before you get started, there are a couple of things we'd like to address in regard to the program.

)) **Training frequency:** Although there are three workouts in this phase, it doesn't necessarily mean you'll be training three times per week. Some weeks you will, but due to the heavy nervous system demand, we want you to think not in terms of a calendar week, but rather how many days recovery you'll need between workouts. Therefore, in this phase, you'll be training every third day in an effort to ensure adequate nervous system recovery. So if you do Workout A on a Monday, you may not do Workout B until Thursday. The next workout would then follow on Sunday, and so on. This means instead of 4 weeks or 28 days, this program will take you 34 days to complete. Believe us, you'll need the extra rest if you're doing it right (i.e., with very high intensity and gut-busting effort).

)) **Warming up:** When you're lifting as heavy as you will be in this phase, you don't just jump into it cold. You need to make sure that you're properly warmed up. Now mind you, we're not talking about 5-minutes-on-the-stationary-bike warmed up. That's fine for raising body temperature and increasing bloodflow to the muscles, but you're also going to need a neural warmup. It's important that you do a couple of light sets of increasing load to get your muscles and nervous system accustomed to the movement pattern and progressive loading of the exercises you'll be doing during your workout. This need not be a long, drawn-out process. All you need are three or four warmup sets of increasing weight to adequately prepare you to lift.

Let's say, for example, that you were doing Workout A. After a quick 5-minute generalized warmup to get the blood flowing and the appropriate mobility sequence from Chapter 6, you would then proceed to your first lift (Trap Bar Deadlift). Let's also assume for argument's sake that your current 2RM is 315. Begin by doing one set of six reps with just the unloaded bar. This will help set the movement pattern in your head and familiarize your body with the specific task at hand. Now you're ready to load. Immediately upon finishing your last rep, increase the weight to 135 pounds, and do four reps. As soon as you're done, bump it up to 225, and do three reps. After two more reps at 250 pounds, rest a couple of minutes before beginning your first set. The best part about this warmup protocol is that it allows you to avoid the high-rep burnout typical of most warmup protocols. We cringe every time we see a guy do sets of 15, 12, and 10 reps as a prep for going heavy. It's wasted energy, plain and simple.

)) **Progression:** You're going to have to be careful with your weight increases here. While it's important to keep the momentum building from one workout to the next, you don't want to get too aggressive and screw everything up. We suggest making small, manageable increases that basically ensure continued progress. Going back to our previous example using the squat, after achieving a new personal best of 305, your goal for the next

workout probably shouldn't be much higher than 310. So your first wave of your next workout might look something like:

280 × 4

290 × 3

300 × 2

And your second:

290 × 4

300 × 3

310 × 2

Bear in mind, though, that the amount of the weight increase also has a lot to do with where you are in the program. In the early stages of the program, you may find that you can be a little more aggressive with your weight increments. Later on, however, as your body begins to adapt to the workout, you might have to be a bit more judicious when adding weight. It's quite possible that in the first couple of weeks, you might be able to go up as much as 10 to 15 pounds per workout as opposed to just 5. Whatever the case, just do your best to make sure the weight continues to climb for the entire 4 weeks.

Remember, to a lot of you, training for strength is going to be a pretty novel concept. This isn't body building or general fitness training where the goal is to induce fatigue or to give your muscles a really great pump. For this 4-week period, you're going to be training your nervous system to become more efficient at recruiting your muscle fibers to contract. You're also going to be generating a lot more force with those muscles than you're used to. The last thing you need to do here is go into captain cross-trainer mode and try to shorten the rest intervals in the interest of "getting a good workout." Do that and your poundages will surely suffer. So just take your time and stay focused, and we promise you the results will be worth it in the end.

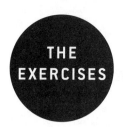

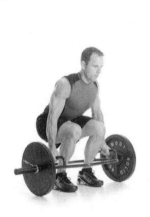

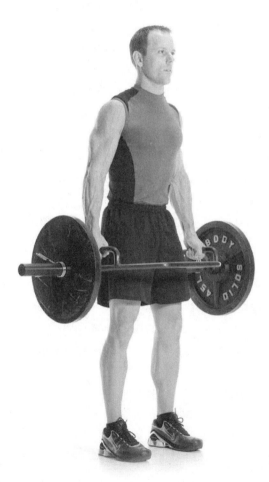

Trap Bar Deadlift

(quads, glutes, hamstrings, lower back, upper back)

Stand inside a trap bar, and squat down to grab the handles. Keep your chest up and your back straight as you drive your feet through the floor to lift the weight off the ground. At the top, your back should be straight, with your hips directly beneath your shoulders. Pause momentarily before lowering the weight back down and repeating the sequence.

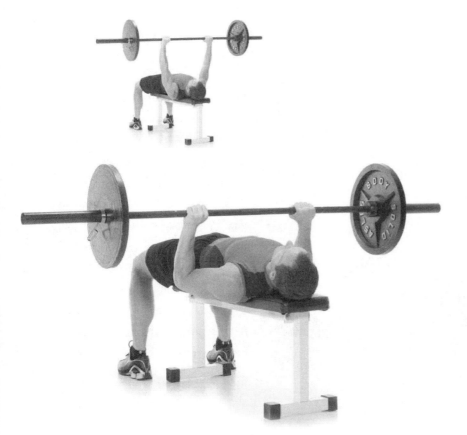

Flat Bench Press
(chest, shoulders, triceps)

Lie on a flat bench underneath a barbell. The bar should be lined up over your face at the start of the lift. Grab the bar with a close (14- to 18-inch) grip, and keep your feet flat on the floor as you lift the weight off the supports. When the weight is lined up over your chest, begin by lowering the bar down to the proper depth (see Chapter 3). Pause at the bottom for a second, and press back up.

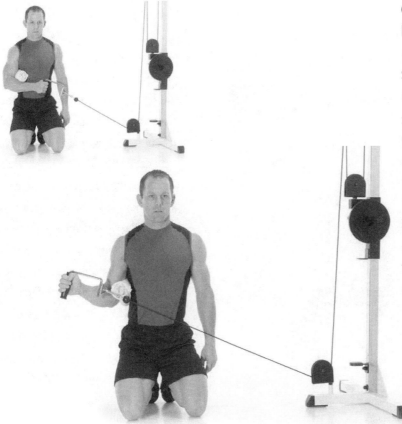

Cable External Rotation
(external rotators)

Stand or kneel sideways to a cable machine with your far arm bent 90 degrees and a rolled-up towel between your elbow and hip. Starting with your arm across your abdominals, externally rotate your forearm by swinging it out and using your elbow as a hinge. Go as far as you can without extending your wrist, and pause there momentarily before slowly returning to the starting position.

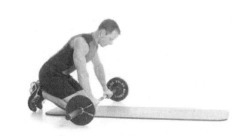

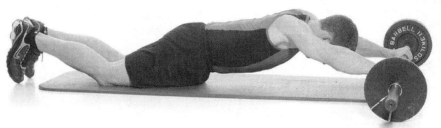

Barbell Rollouts
(abdominals,
lower back, shoulders)

Kneel on an exercise mat behind a barbell with small 5-pound plates at each end. Grab the bar with a shoulder-width grip, and starting with your hands directly beneath your shoulders, slowly allow the bar to roll out as your body travels with it. Allow your arms to go forward over your head, and get your face as close as possible to the floor without allowing your back to round. Once you've reached your farthest point, use your core musculature to bring you back to the starting position.

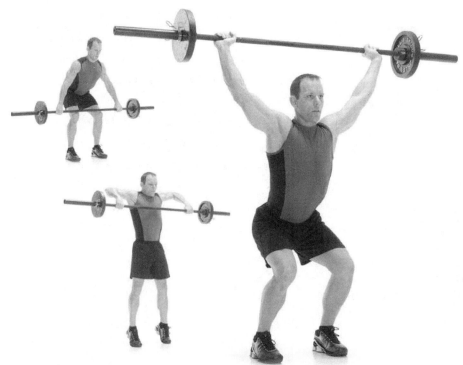

Hang Snatch
(glutes, hamstrings,
quads, lower back,
upper back, trapezius)

Stand the same way you did to begin the clean and press, only this time, use a snatch grip (at least twice shoulder width). Begin the movement the same way as you did the clean, by extending the knees, hips, and ankles and by rapidly shrugging the bar. This time though, "throw" the bar up higher with your arms as straight as possible, and then drop under and catch it while your arms are still straight. In the finish position, the bar will be straight overhead, and you'll be in a half squat position. Flip the bar down, and repeat.

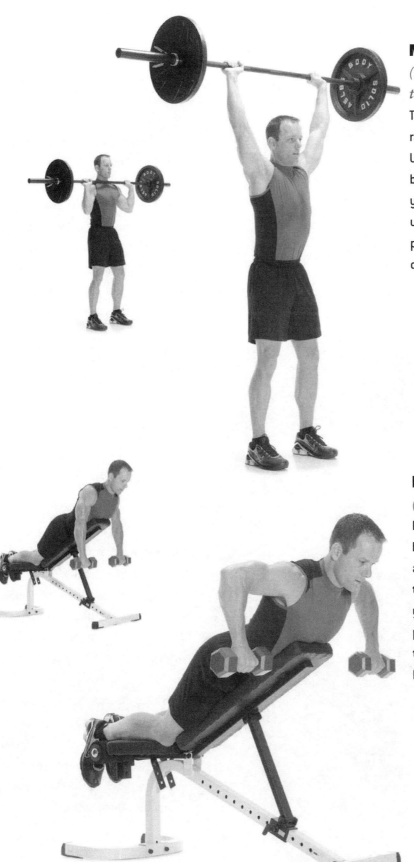

Military Press
(shoulders, trapezius, triceps)

Take a bar off the supports of a squat rack set at about collarbone level. Using a shoulder-width grip, walk the bar back a step or two, and then with your knees slightly bent, press the bar up overhead until your arms are completely straight. Lower the bar back down to chin level, and repeat.

Prone Row
(upper back, biceps)

Lie prone over a 45-degree incline bench holding a couple of dumbbells at arm's length. With your palms positioned so they face behind you, pinch your shoulder blades together, and pull the weights up to the sides of your torso. Hold for a second, and lower back to the starting position.

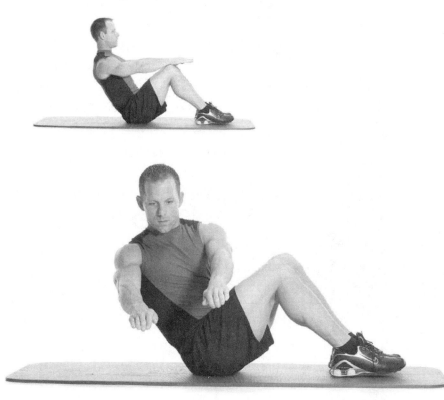

Russian Twists

(abdominals, obliques, lower back)

Sit on the floor with your knees bent and your feet flat, and lean back with your arms outstretched over your knees. Without moving your legs, rotate as far as you can to one side and then back to the center before repeating to the other side. Remember to pull your belly button in toward your spine throughout the exercise. For added difficulty, use light weights.

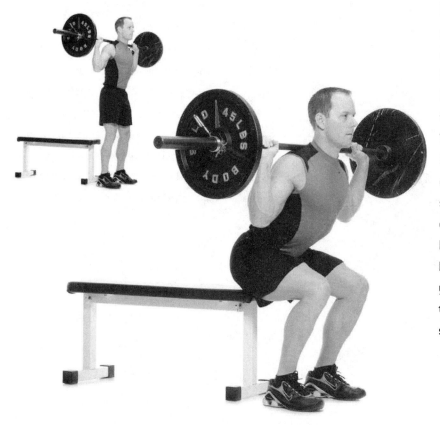

Box Squat

(glutes, hamstrings, quads, erectors)

Walk into a squat rack, and place a loaded barbell across your back near the bottom of your shoulder blades. Walk back out until you're straddling a bench or sturdy box you've placed a couple of steps behind you. Your toes should be turned out, with your feet out wide to the sides of the box. Begin by driving the hips back and then bending the knees until you lower yourself to the point where your hips touch the box. Pause there for a second, and stand back up.

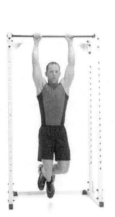

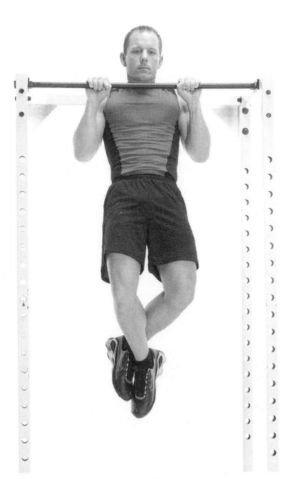

Pullups

(upper back, biceps, brachialis)

Grab an overhead bar with a shoulder-width, pronated grip. From a dead hang, pull yourself up until your chin clears the bar or your chest touches it.

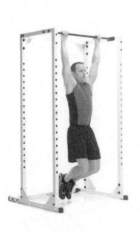

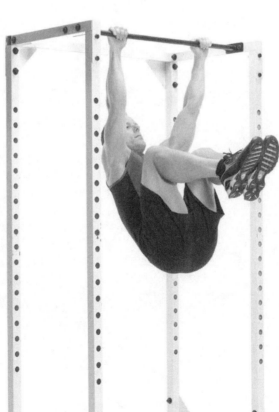

Hanging Leg Raise

(abdominals, obliques)

Grab an overhead bar with a shoulder-width pronated grip. From a dead hang, proceed to lift your legs up toward your chest until your body folds in half. This can be done with either bent knees or straight legs if you have the strength. Just be sure that the knee angle remains constant throughout the exercise. No swinging or jerking your way up.

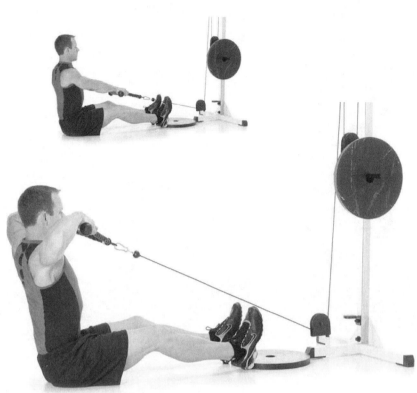

Cable Rows to Neck, with a rope handle

(rear deltoids, upper trapezius, biceps)

Sit at a cable row station, and grasp the rope handle at each end. With your torso perfectly upright over your hips, pull the rope back, keeping your elbows away from your sides, so your elbows finish up near your ears. Lower the weight back to the starting position, and repeat.

STRONG WORDS

If you execute this phase properly, your body will be primed and ready to put on some serious muscle in Phase IV. Your increased strength and improved neurological efficiency will have you absolutely manhandling weights you used to consider heavy. As long as you continue to provide your body with the rest and nutritional support it needs, you should be positively thrilled with your results when you've finished the program. For now, though, just focus on getting as strong as you possibly can.

When it's all said and done, you will have built yourself a tremendous strength base from which to progress. And, despite the fact that is far from a traditional hypertrophy phase, because the loads are so heavy, don't be surprised if you end up sporting a little extra muscle mass courtesy of all that extra attention you've paid to those oft-ignored type IIb fibers. Besides which, throw in the steady flow of quality nutrients you'll be ingesting on a daily basis and your body will have no choice but to start sprouting muscle all over the place. The cool part is: You'll now have the strength to go along with all that muscle. That's something that even the most dedicated "bodybuilders" often can't lay claim to.

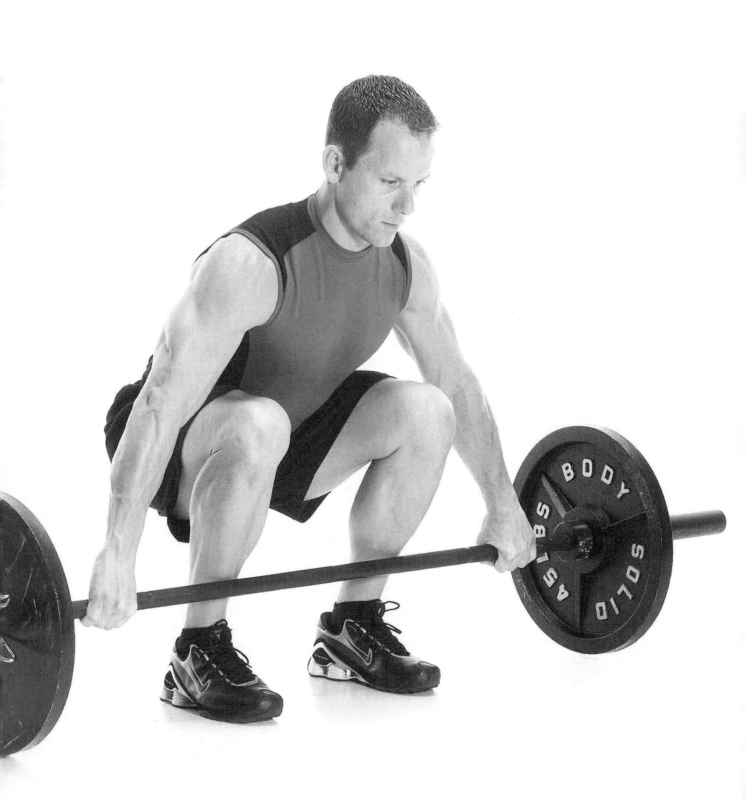

TRAINING: PHASE IV

>> It took you a while, but you finally got here. After weeks of unfamiliar exercises and seemingly bizarre set and rep schemes, you're about to experience a little normalcy. No more feeling like that one kid who's different from the others. For the next 4 weeks, you'll actually be doing workouts that are at least somewhat similar to what everyone else is doing. You don't have to feel like you're chained to the squat rack or can't go beyond five reps per set. This phase is all about harnessing the improvements you've made over the past 12 weeks into one extremely comprehensive muscle-building bonanza! Prepare yourself, though; this one is going to be different from all the others—a lot different.

The first major difference you're going to notice is in regards to your training frequency. For the first time since you embarked on this little journey, you're going to be lifting four times per week on a split routine, whereby you work both your upper and lower body twice every 7 days. We know, we know, this is akin to sacrilege in some hardgainer circles, but as you've probably guessed by now, there's a method to our madness. Although your training frequency will be somewhat high, the volume will be relatively low (12 to 14 total sets per workout), enabling you to get into and out of the gym fairly quickly. Considering the relative brevity of the workouts and superior nutritional support you're now supplying your body with, this increase in training volume won't be a problem for a short time frame.

The other big difference is that you'll be working with a variety of loads in each workout. Unlike previous phases where you stuck predominantly with either light (Phase I) or heavy loads (Phases II and III), this phase mixes the loading for the ultimate muscle-building stimulus. You'll do some heavy, low-rep work to maintain strength and stimulate those powerful fast-twitch muscle fibers as well as some more moderate-load training to target your type IIa fibers. As you may remember from our little physiology lesson in Chapter 4, your type IIa fibers possess both strength and endurance properties.

They're also the ones that bear the brunt of the stress when doing more traditional bodybuilding-style workouts. And although they don't contribute much to overall strength development, they can help improve the appearance of your muscles to a substantial degree.

Confused? We thought perhaps you might be. After all, how can a muscle, or group of muscles, improve visual appeal and not experience an accompanying increase in strength? The same way that most bodybuilders look bigger and more muscular than powerlifters but often aren't anywhere near as strong. Bodybuilders spend the bulk of their time working with moderate loads and higher reps, placing much more stress on their type IIa fibers. That's all well and good since these muscles do have a decent capacity for growth. The only trouble is, some scientists believe that much of the growth that does occur takes place in portions of the muscle cell that have nothing to do with making it contract. This growth between the muscle fibers serves to increase the muscle's size without necessarily improving its ability to generate force. So although the muscles do get bigger, they don't necessarily get any stronger.

So why should you care about this stuff? Because when your goal is to get bigger, you need to maximize the growth potential of *all* your muscle fibers. So what if higher rep training doesn't contribute much to increasing strength? You're looking to put on some size, plain and simple! If the area surrounding a muscle fiber can account for roughly 25 to 30 percent of that muscle's size, why would you want to leave that untapped? Besides, it's not like you're totally abandoning all strength work. You'll still begin each workout with some heavy-load work; you're just throwing in some lighter weights to cover all your bases.

Before you get started with the actual workouts, here are a few little tips to help you along the way.

》 **Exercise pairings/rest intervals:** Most of the exercises featured in this phase have been paired into supersets of opposing muscle actions, although there are some pairings that blast some of the same muscles consecutively (i.e., Snatch Grip Deadlifts and Glute Ham Raises). Whenever you see two exercises that share the same letter of the alphabet, they are to be performed one right after the other with no rest. After you have performed the second exercise, you can then rest for a length of time commensurate with the load that was used. After Workout A supersets, rest 2 to 3 minutes; after Workout B supersets, rest 1 to 2 minutes; and after Workout C supersets, rest 60 to 90 seconds. After completing the rest interval, go back to the first exercise in that same pairing, and continue until you have completed the desired number of sets before moving on to the next pairing.

》 **Supplemental activity:** More so than any other phase thus far, your objective during this 4-week period is to build muscle. In addition to making sure you're eating enough calories to support growth, during this phase, you must also be extremely careful with supplemental physical activity. There's nothing wrong with throwing in a cardio workout or two each week, so long as you're covering the additional caloric expenditure and keeping them as far removed from your weight workouts as possible. Just be sure to keep them short and sweet and of an intensity high enough to offer a potent cardiovascular stimulus in as short a time frame as possible (see Chapter 5 for cardio workouts designed to complement this phase).

》 **Warmups:** You can still employ the same type of general warmup and dynamic flexibility of the previous phases. You may also want to go through the same neural warmup featured in the previous chapter as a means of preparing for the heavy lifts that kick off each workout. After that, however, you're best off just going straight into the other exercises, since the loads will be relatively light.

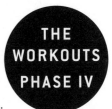
The workouts in this section differ from those in previous phases in two ways: First of all, you'll be lifting four times per week (two upper body and two lower body workouts), and secondly, you will be supersetting all of the exercises. This is why the exercises are broken down into groups using numbers and letters. For example, you would do a set of the A-1 exercise and then immediately proceed to the A-2 exercise before taking a 90-second rest. You would then continue with this sequence until you have performed the desired number of sets for that pairing. Then you would proceed on to B-1, B-2, and so on.

UPPER BODY: MONDAY AND FRIDAY

WORKOUT A

EXERCISE	SETS/REPS
1. Close Grip Incline Bench Press	3 × 4–5
2. Sternum Pullup	3 × 4–5*
1. Reverse Pushups (feet elevated)	3 × 4–5*
2. Incline Dumbbell Press	3 × 4–5

WORKOUT B

EXERCISE	SETS/REPS
1. Telle Flys	2 × 6–10
2. Bent Over Row	2 × 6–10
1. Swiss Ball Shoulder Press	2 × 6–10
2. High Pulls	2 × 6–10

WORKOUT C

EXERCISE	SETS/REPS
1. Hammer Curl & Press	2 × 10–12
2. Pullover Triceps Extension	2 × 10–12
1. Reverse Flys	2 × 10–12
2. Cross Body Cable External Rotation	2 × 10–12

LOWER BODY: TUESDAY AND SATURDAY

WORKOUT A

EXERCISE	SETS/REPS
1. Front Squat	3 × 4–5
2. Negative Leg Curl	3 × 4–5
1. Snatch Grip Deadlift***	3 × 4–5
2. Glute Ham Raises	3 × 4–5

WORKOUT B

EXERCISE	SETS/REPS
1. Lunges	2 × 6–10**
2. Weighted Back Extension	2 × 6–10
1. Barbell Hack Squat	2 × 6–10
2. Standing Calf Raise	2 × 6–10

WORKOUT C

EXERCISE	SETS/REPS
1. Cable Woodchopper	2 × 10–12
2. Swiss Ball Crunch	2 × 10–12
1. Slant Board Reverse Crunch	2 × 10–12
2. Saxon Side Bends	2 × 10–12

  * Add extra weight if necessary.

 ** Indicates number of reps to be performed on each side.

*** Those lacking adequate flexibility can opt for the Trap Bar Deadlift done off 25-pound plates.

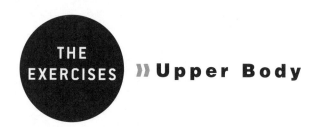

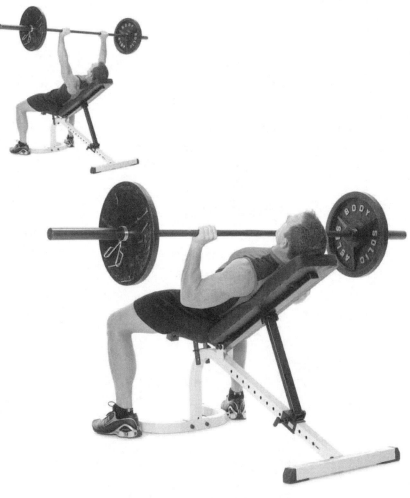

Close Grip Incline Bench Press

(chest, front delts, triceps)

Lie on your back on an incline bench, and grasp the barbell with a close (14- to 18-inch) grip. Lift the bar off the supports, and lower it toward your collarbone to the appropriate depth (see Chapter 3), being sure to keep your elbows in fairly close to your body. Pause for a second, then press back up.

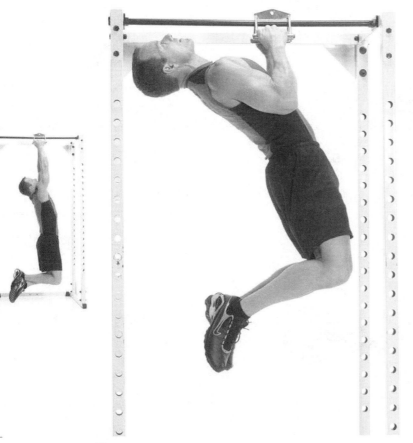

Sternum Pullup
(upper back, biceps)

This exercise is best done with a semi-supinated, or neutral grip (palms facing each other), but if you don't have access to these kinds of handles, a regular bar will work, if you have the strength. Grasp an overhead bar with a pronated grip. Starting from a dead hang, pull yourself up toward the bar while simultaneously driving your hips forward and leaning back as shown. In the top position, your body should be at a 45-degree angle to the floor with your chest out and shoulder blades pulled back. Lower, and repeat.

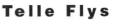

Telle Flys
(chest, front delts, triceps)

We got this one from renowned trainer Jerry Telle, who specializes in increasing the muscular overload of an exercise. To begin, select a weight that is substantially heavier than you normally use to do dumbbell flys (if you usually use 20s, try 40s instead). Next, lie back on a bench, and press the dumbbells up into position over your chest. Now, bend your elbows slightly, and work the weights down in a wide, arcing motion. When your arms are even with the level of the bench, bring the dumbbells in toward your chest by bending your elbows and pressing them back up.

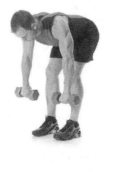

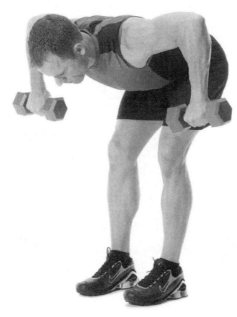

Bent Over Row
(upper back, biceps)

Hold a barbell or a pair of dumbbells with a pronated shoulders-width grip. Next, bend your knees slightly and lean over at the waist until your torso is almost parallel to the floor. Being sure to maintain a slight arch in your lower back, pinch your shoulder blades together as you pull the weights up until your elbows pass your torso. Hold for a second, lower, and repeat.

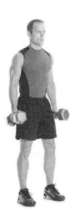

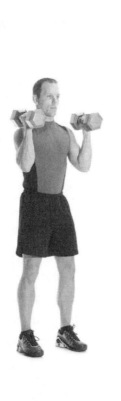

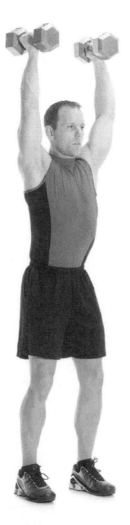

Hammer Curl & Press
(brachioradialis, biceps, shoulders and triceps)

Stand holding a pair of dumbbells at your sides with a semi-supinated grip. Begin by curling the dumbbells up toward your shoulders. Once there, press the dumbbells up overhead. Lower, and repeat.

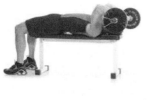

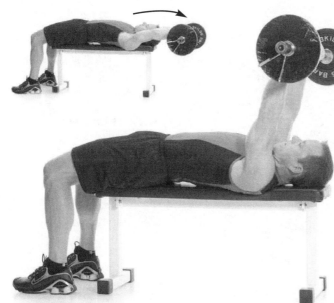

Pullover Triceps Extension
(lats, chest, triceps)

Lie back on an exercise bench holding a barbell (or two dumbbells) at arm's length over your chest. Begin by keeping your upper arms still and lowering the barbell toward the crown of your head. Once there, maintain the same degree of bend in the elbows, and arc the bar back down and toward the floor until your arms are about even with your ears. Pause momentarily, and then work the weight back up to the crown of the head, and extend your arms to finish the repetition.

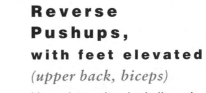

Reverse Pushups,
with feet elevated
(upper back, biceps)

Lie underneath a barbell set in the supports in the squat rack at about waist height. Grasp the bar with a false grip; place your feet up on a bench (or Swiss Ball) that's in front of you. Next, lift your hips, so your body forms a straight line, and with your elbows held out to the sides, pull yourself up toward the bar. At the top, your chest should be as close to the bar as possible. Lower yourself until your arms are straight, and repeat.

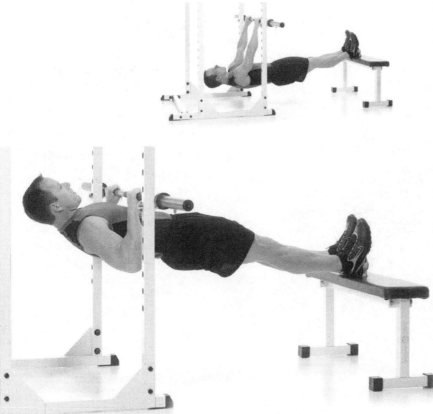

141

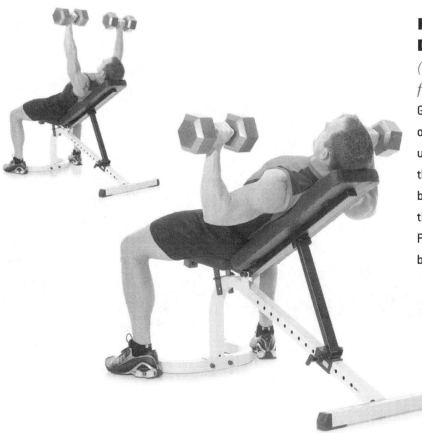

Incline Dumbbell Press
(chest, front deltoids, triceps)

Grab a pair of dumbbells, and lie back on a flat bench. Press the dumbbells up, so they're right over your chest at the start. Begin by lowering the dumbbells down toward your chest until they reach the appropriate depth. Pause for a second, and press them back up.

Swiss Ball Shoulder Press
(deltoids, triceps, core)

Sit on a Swiss Ball with your knees at a 90-degree angle and a pair of dumbbells in line with your cheekbones as shown. Without losing your balance, press the weights overhead, and then slowly lower them back down.

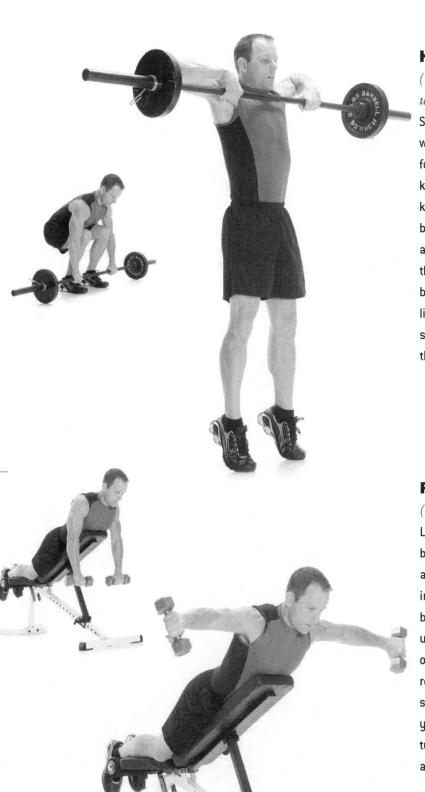

High Pulls

*(trapezius,
upper back, biceps)*

Stand holding a barbell with a shoulder-width, pronated grip, leaning slightly forward so the bar is in line with your knees. Begin by extending the hips, knees, and ankles to accelerate the bar up as you simultaneously shrug and pull the weight up to your chest. In the top position, you should be on the balls of your feet with the barbell in line with your chest. Hold for a split second, and lower the weight back to the starting position.

Reverse Flys

(upper back, rear deltoids)

Lie prone over a 45-degree exercise bench holding a pair of dumbbells at arm's length. Keeping a slight bend in your elbows, pinch your shoulder blades together, and work your arms up in a wide, arcing motion. At the top of the movement, your elbows should remain slightly bent, and you should see the weights out of the corners of your eyes. Use a pronated grip as pictured here for increased rear shoulder activation.

143

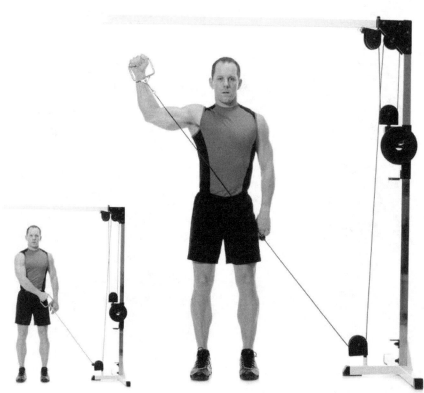

Cross Body Cable External Rotation

(external rotators)

Stand sideways to a cable station with a low handle attachment. Reach across your body, and grab the low handle. With the working hand in front of your opposite pocket, rotate your arm up and out as shown so that your arm ends up over your head on the opposite side of your body and your palm is now facing forward. Lower, and repeat.

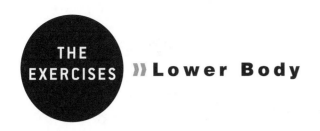

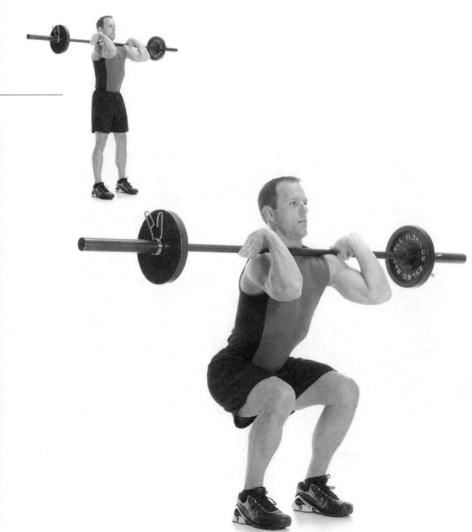

Front Squat

(quads, glutes, hamstrings, upper back)

Walk into a squat rack with a barbell set at about collarbone level. Next, rest the bar on the meaty portion of the front deltoids with the bar lightly touching your throat. Once you've supported the bar, walk back a few steps, and set your feet slightly wider than shoulder width apart. Next, begin the movement by breaking at the knee first, then the hips, and maintain an arch in your lower back.

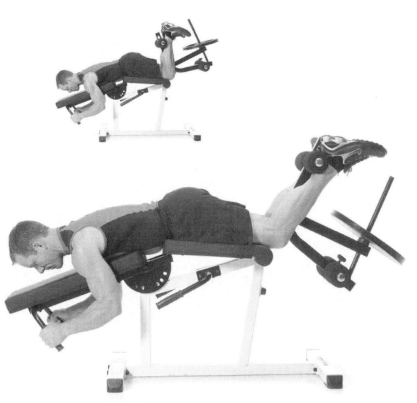

Negative Leg Curl

(hamstrings, calves)

Lie on a leg curl machine with your knees hanging off the pad and your feet flexed (toes pulled toward your shins). Use your hamstrings and calves to pull the weight up toward your rear end, being sure to avoid thrusting the weight up. At the top of the movement, point your toes, and lower the weight using only your hamstrings.

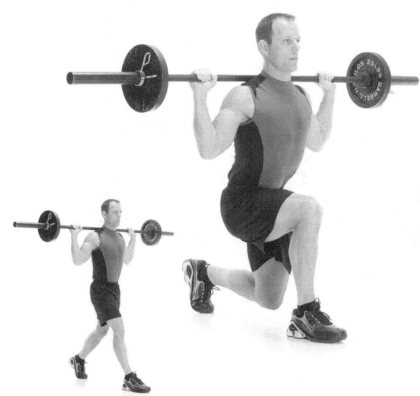

Lunges

(quads, glutes, hamstrings)

Stand holding either a pair of dumbbells or a barbell across your shoulders. Next, take a large step forward (2 ½ to 3 feet in front of you), and bend both knees as you lower your hips down and slightly forward. Once you've reached the bottom position where the lead leg is parallel to the floor, immediately push back up to the starting position. Repeat with other leg.

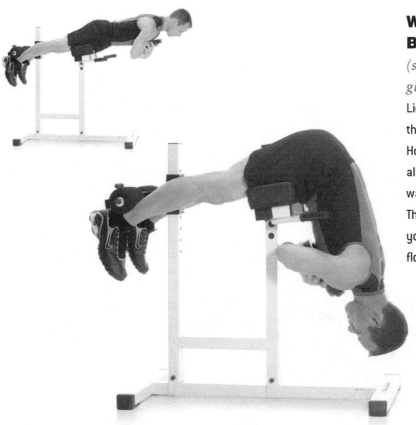

Weighted Back Extension

(spinal erectors, glutes, hamstrings)

Lie prone with your feet hooked under the foot supports of a Roman chair. Holding a weigh across your chest, allow your body to bend forward at the waist, and round your back slightly. Then extend yourself back up until your torso is just past parallel to the floor.

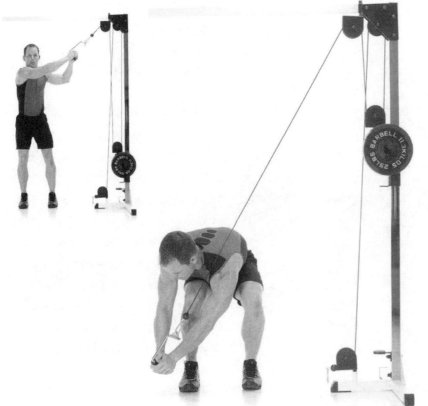

Cable Woodchopper

(abdominals, obliques)

Stand sideways to a cable station holding the high handle over one shoulder with both hands. With your knees bent and your torso facing straight ahead, begin by torquing at the hips and midsection to accelerate the bar down and across your body until you finish with your hands outside your opposite calf.

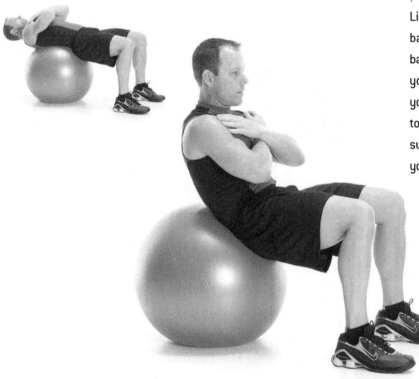

Swiss Ball Crunch

(abdominals)

Lie back on a Swiss Ball, allowing your back to conform to the shape of the ball. With your feet flat on the floor and your knees bent 90 degrees, keep your hips still as you raise your upper torso off the surface of the ball. Be sure to round your spine and crunch your rib cage down toward your pelvis.

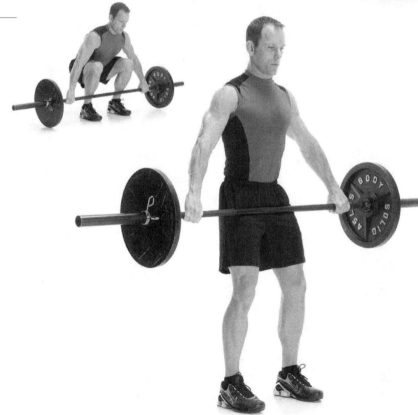

Snatch Grip Deadlift

(glutes, hamstrings, spinal erectors)

Stand over a loaded barbell with your feet about shoulder width apart. Next, bend over, and grasp the bar with a "snatch" grip (about twice shoulder width). Get your hips low, and try to keep your torso as upright as possible. (You will need to bend over substantially.) Keeping your arms straight, drive your feet through the floor, and extend your hips up and forward to stand with the weight. Lower the weights back until they touch the floor, and repeat.

Glute Ham Raise

(glutes, hamstrings, spinal erectors)

Two options here: an actual Glute Ham Bench or a "natural" Glute Ham Raise. Bench: Position yourself on the bench with your feet against the footplate and thighs on the pad. Lying face down with arms folded across your chest, begin by extending your spine and then bending your knees to pull your torso back toward your feet. Natural: Using a partner or heavy object to anchor your calves, place a towel under your knees, and lower your body toward the floor. Get as close as you can, and either use your glutes and hamstrings to lift you back up, or drop the last few inches to the floor, and do a pushup to get to the point where your lower body can pull you up.

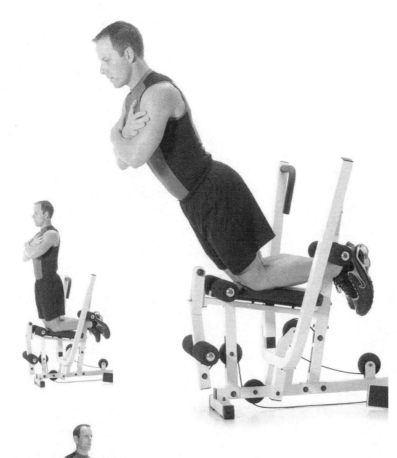

Barbell Hack Squat

(quads, glutes, hamstrings)

Set up a pair of 25-pound plates about a foot behind the supports of a squat rack. With the bar set at about hip level, stand in front of it, and grab it with a shoulder-width grip behind your back. Next, slowly walk back toward the weight plates until you've got both your heels elevated up on the plates. Keeping your back as straight as possible, break at the knees first, and descend into as deep a squat as you can. When you've reached your lowest point, drive your feet into the floor to stand back up to the starting position.

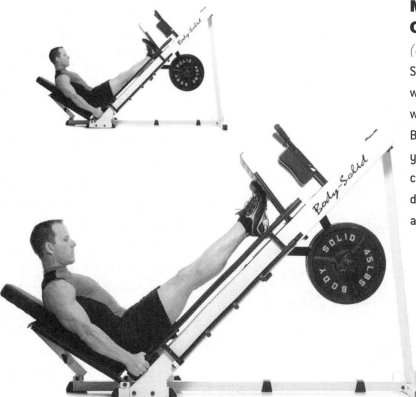

Machine Calf Raise
(calves)

Sit in an angled leg press machine with only the balls of your feet on the weight plate and your legs straight. Begin by letting the weight sled give you a good stretch by letting your toes come down toward you. Then reverse direction and push the sled up as high as you can. Lower and repeat.

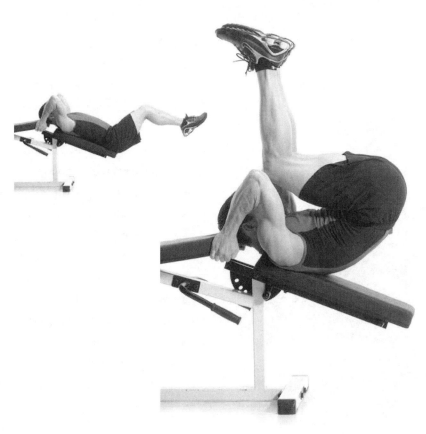

Slant Board Reverse Crunch
(abdominals)

Lie back on a slant board set at about a 45- to 60-degree angle. Holding on to the top of the board, begin with your knees stacked right over your hips. Using your abdominals, fold your legs back toward your chest until your tailbone comes slightly off the board. Lower, and repeat.

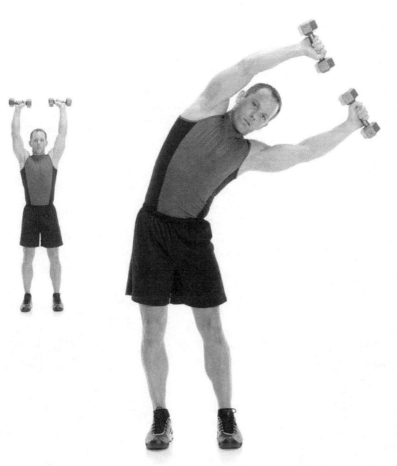

Saxon Side Bends

(obliques)

Stand with your feet about shoulder width apart, holding a pair of light dumbbells with your palms facing forward. Keeping your lower body perfectly still, lean as far as you can to one side without twisting your torso in any way. Once you've gone as far as you can, use your obliques to get back to the starting position.

SHORT AND SWEET

Once again, you're probably going to be surprised by the relative brevity of your workouts during this phase. Those of you who are used to the high-volume approach to strength training will be tempted to do more. We strongly advise against this! The only way a guy in your situation is going to make progress training four times per week is if the workouts are kept quick and intense. Start adding extra exercises and sets, and you'll be completely defeating the purpose. So please, for your own sake, resist the urge to play mad scientist. Leave that to us.

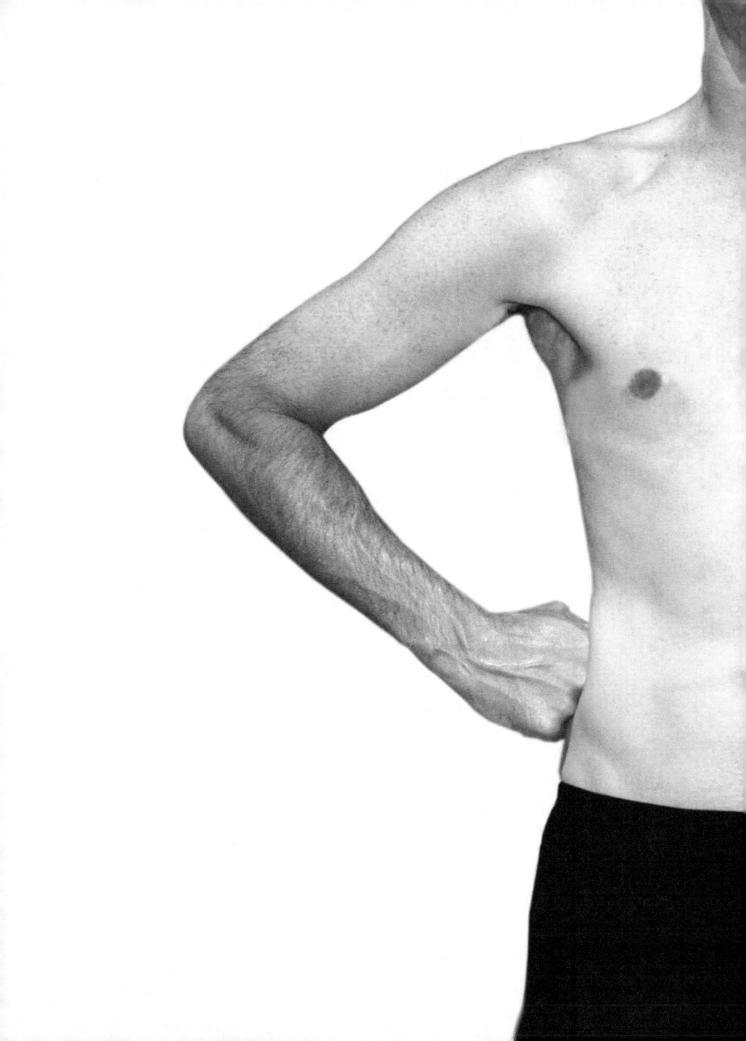

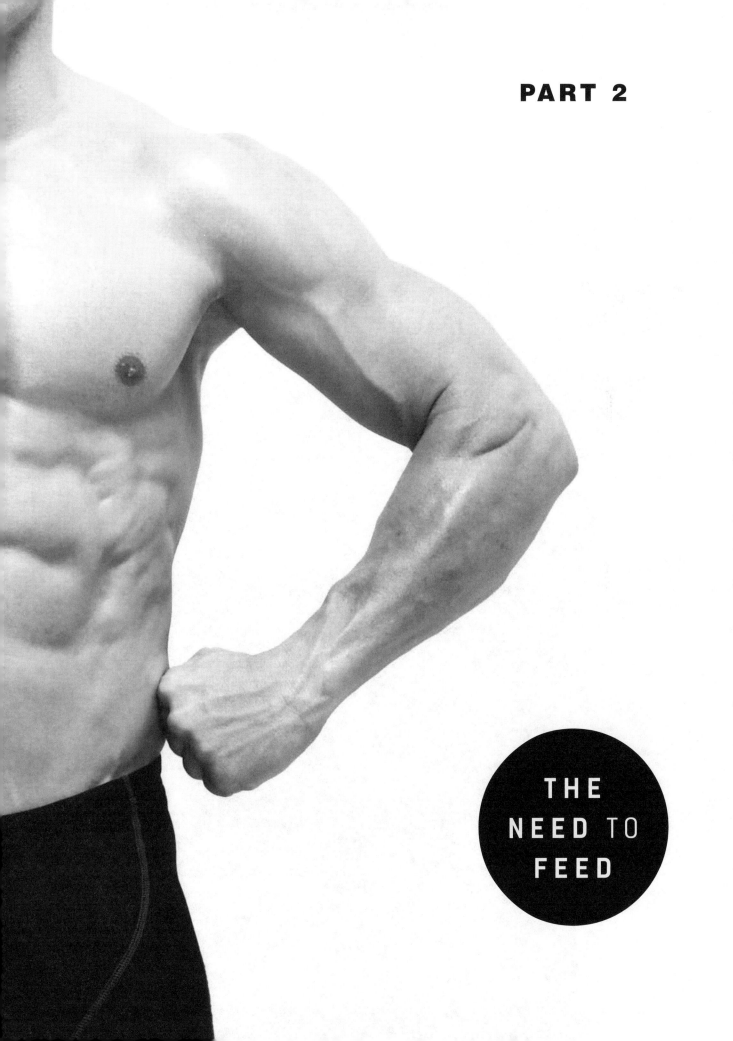

PART 2

THE
NEED TO
FEED

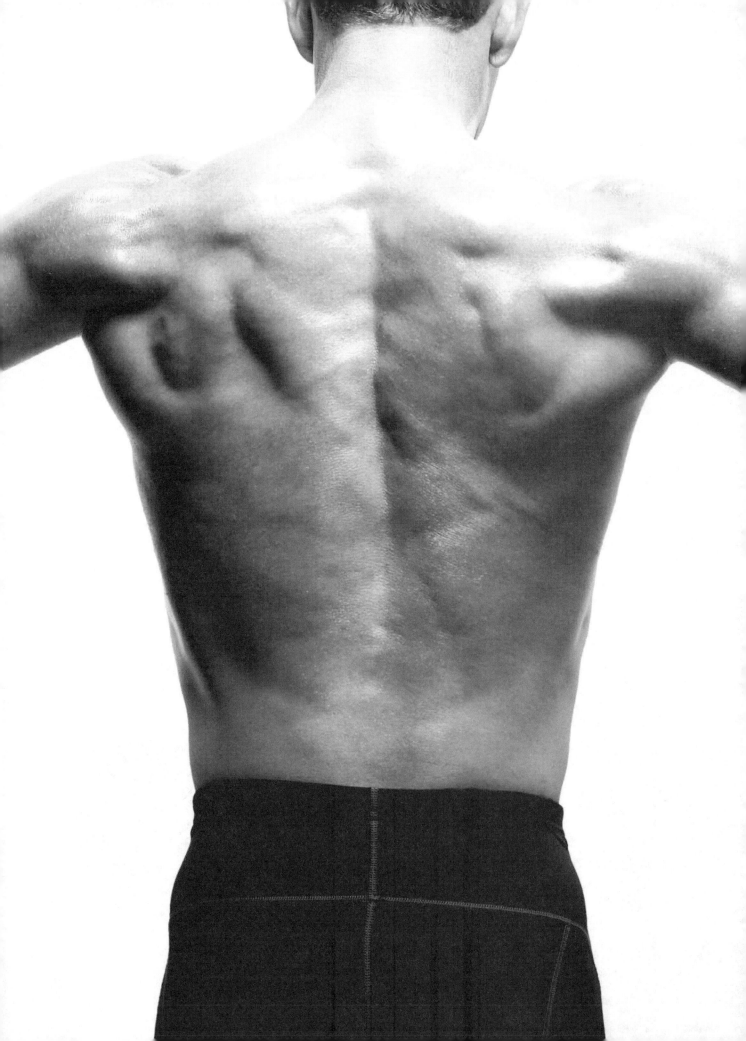

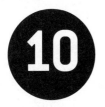

INTRODUCTORY NUTRITION FOR THE HYPERTROPHY-CHALLENGED

In the introduction to this book, Mike Mejia called you Gumby. Me, I'm not so insensitive. After all, just because you're so skinny that you actually have to jump around in the shower to get wet doesn't mean you need to be the subject of my ridicule. Heck no, it's not your fault that when you turn to the side and stick out your tongue, you look like a zipper!

Or is it?

In this book, we provide a justification for why certain individuals, those we call *hypertrophy-challenged*, may have a hard time gaining muscle strength and mass. And if you've read carefully, you've noticed that a lot of it has to do with things that are often out of your control, things subject to genetic influences such as hormonal status, muscle-fiber type, biomechanical disadvantages, metabolic challenges, etc. However, it's about time for a big reality check—this check being drafted against a huge scientific bank account. According to what we currently know about genes and their expression, sorry, you can't blame your genes alone for your lack of progress in the gym. Rather, you must look within, literally.

Look deep within the cells of your body, and you'll find the center of your physiological universe, the cell nucleus. Inside the nucleus, you'll find your genetic code, a series of molecules that provides a blueprint for who you are. These molecules, your genes, told your body how to develop when you were nothing more than a fertilized egg—so it's a good thing that your genes weren't scrambled. And nowadays, since you're all grown, the genes tell your cells how to divide, how to heal, how to respond to exercise, how to metabolize the food you eat, and how to remember the words you're reading right now. So it would be safe to say that your genetic makeup is pretty important. In the science world, we describe this genetic makeup as your *genotype*. Remember that word.

At this point, after presenting the laundry list of what genes are responsible for, it may seem as if genes alone control your fate. But don't send any hate mail to Mom and Dad, please. Have you heard of the word *phenotype*? Scientifically speaking, we use this word to describe the attributes of an organism. In your case, your eye color is a phenotype. Your height is also a phenotype. And your body-fat percentage is another phenotype. With two new words—genotype and phenotype—under your belt, let's figure out the relationship between the two.

The expression of a few traits, such as eye color, is the result of a certain genetic switch that was flipped during gestation, handing you your set of baby blues (or browns or greens). If you like your eye color, send Mom flowers and Dad a tie since this trait is 100 percent their doing. Your height, like your eye color, was also largely determined by your genetics. However, nutrition, activity, hormonal status, and a few other environmental factors could have played a small role in whether or not you came up short. Unlike eye color and height, though, when it comes to muscle mass and body composition, what you look like, your phenotype, is determined by the interplay between your genotype *and* your environment. Of course, your genotype, that's fixed. But thank the heavens above; your environment is under your control. In fact, according to two research studies, one published in the *Annals of Human Biology* and the other in *Human Heredity,* about 50 to 60 percent of your somatotype (whether you're of the ectomorphic, mesomorphic, or endomorphic persuasion) can be accounted for by the genes passed down from your parents. The other 40 to 50 percent just so happens to be environmentally influenced.

So, looking back at the original question, is it your fault that you have a hard time putting on muscle, a hard time getting in your best shape ever, a hard time going from Scrawny to Brawny? The answer is probably yes. In some ways, it is. Although your genes might be presenting some serious challenges to loading up those bones with muscle, everyone can currently see those bones because you haven't imposed the right environment to alter that hypertrophy-challenged, ectomorphic phenotype. If you want the muscle badly enough, no matter how ecto-, endo-, or meso- morphed-up you are, if you make some serious lifestyle changes, you'll get it. That's right, even if you've tried all the *Muscle and Fitness* magazine workouts, experimented with all the protein supplements you can stomach, and followed the advice of countless "experts," there's still hope.

Of course, with all the nasty-tasting amino acid tablets out there, there's yet another bitter pill for you to swallow. The reality is that if you can't seem to reach your physique goals, it's not because your Momma cursed you but because *you've* fallen short in some way. However, don't beat yourself up too much. Your previous attempts at gaining muscle may have failed for one of a number of reasons.

1. Your efforts lacked consistency: For starters, you might not have wholeheartedly committed to making a change in your environment. You might be eating well and training hard only part of the time, quickly becoming demotivated by the apparent lack of progress. Let me tell you this: If you're hypertrophy-challenged, there is no eating well or training hard part of the time. It's all or scrawny, baby. A wise man once said: "Consistency, not novelty, is the secret to uncommon results." Oh wait . . . never mind; John said that.

2. Your efforts lacked intensity: Alternatively, you might have been consistent with your training and nutrition but not really training as hard as you should have or eating as much food as you needed to grow. As with most things in life, commitment takes you beyond the average. But simply showing up is not enough. Without a real focus and desire for success, you won't make the strides you might have otherwise made. Again, with the hypertrophy-challenged, it's train big, eat big, or remain small.

3. You were misinformed: Finally, you might have been committed, consistent, and diligent but had simply been using the wrong "expert" advice. Of course, this is the worst position to be in since the failure wasn't yours alone. Part of the failure can be chalked up to a previous suboptimal coach. So that's why we're here, to eliminate the need for you to seek any other advice outside of this comprehensive muscle-building manual. There are enough people out there who think we're the right coaches to get the job done. Need proof? Well, a group of very intelligent book people and editors let us write this book. Go figure!

In the end, regardless of the reason why you've not achieved your goals, it's time for you to do two things.

1. You need to accept the reality that you're not doomed to a muscle-free existence.

2. You need to accept personal responsibility for adopting the principles in this book and employing them to change your muscle-building environment from a T. S. Eliot–inspired Wasteland to a Fertile Crescent of muscularity.

Now, for those of you new to the game—you young guys and girls or you older guys and gals being introduced to the iron game for the first time—you might still be wet behind the ears and optimistic about your potential. That's good. Optimism is the cornerstone of all successful attempts at progress. So stay optimistic about your potential because, whether you're new to the game or an old grizzled veteran, you're not doomed to your genetics. Rather, your muscle-building environment determines your physique. That's right; environment is a huge part of determining your phenotype. It is your key to making progress in and outside of the gym. Environment is what allows you to no longer be a slave to your genetics. And of course, when it comes to building muscle, the most important part of your environment is nutrition.

I've said it a thousand times before, if I've said it once: Many guys and girls we meet aren't hardgainers at all; they're simply undereaters. That's right; those individuals out there lamenting their cursed genetics might not even be hypertrophy-challenged at all. Instead, they might simply be a few dozen meals away from being their gym's equivalent of Adonis. But regardless of whether you're an ectomorph or hungry mesomorph, if you want to pack on the lean mass, getting your nutrition straight shall become your foremost concern. Bathing your muscles with micronutrients (vitamins and minerals), macronutrients (carbohydrates, proteins, and fats), and energy (calories) is the best way to create that well-muscled phenotype you're after.

Before we get to the nutrition chapters though, we need to be clear on a few things. First, most people, based on their own past experiences, usually have some internal notion of how much food should be enough, how many calories they should try to eat, and how much protein, carbohydrate, and fat is too much, and this notion stands between them and the body they want. So right now, we want you to remove all such notions from your mind! We're serious. These notions you have probably aren't grounded in reality. Instead, they're probably just arbitrarily based on what you've seen coworkers, gymmates, or professional athletes eat or claim to eat.

Listen up—and listen good because this might be one of the most important lessons for you to take from this book—*changing your physique is an outcome-based pursuit*. This means that you *must* alter your environment, measure the outcome of that alteration, and use the outcome to determine the future changes necessary. Just following a program because it's supposed to work is what fools do. Following a program beyond its effectiveness is a fool's work also. We're in the business of teaching a different approach.

Eating more than before yet not getting bigger? Then increase your food intake again! Eating more than you think you should be eating but still not getting bigger? Keep increasing. When you were practicing for your driver's license test, would you have decided to only practice driving for 1 hour per day regardless of whether you were improving or not? Heck no! You would have practiced for as long as it took to improve enough to get that damn license. Use this same practice in your nutrition, and you're already ahead of 80 percent of the people out there struggling to pack on the pounds. In other words, your success is directly related to your figuring out how much you need to eat to grow.

Secondly, banish all ideas that eating healthy and eating for muscle size are one and the same. Sometimes, unfortunately, these two can be quite exclusive. Now, I'm going to have to be careful to clarify that the nutrition plans presented in the following chapters are designed to promote both health *and* muscle growth. But not all plans out there accomplish both. Some meal plans are awesome for

making you healthier, but they won't do a thing about those protruding ribs or a protruding gut. Other meal plans are awesome for making you bigger or leaner but can actually reduce the quality of your health. So get clear on the fact that just because you eat healthy doesn't mean that you're doing all it takes to get that hard-to-gain muscle mass. If you make this mistake, as others do, you deserve to continue resembling that celery stick you had with lunch. So make no mistake about it; we're not just a couple of muscle heads who are going to teach you how to bulk up, health be damned. Rather, the meal plans in this book achieve the intersection of eating for health and eating for improved muscle mass. Eating as we suggest will help you pack on the pounds while improving your health.

So why do we emphasize these last two points? Well, because we've seen them stand in the way of progress, not only the progress of our clients but also our own progress. Take John, for example; once upon a time, he sat where you're sitting, thinking he was also hypertrophy-challenged. After 2 years of training, at 5'8", he had managed to hit only an embarrassing 150 pounds at 10 percent body fat; his main goal was to bench press his own body weight. Of course, despite his inability to change his environment appropriately, he thought he was doing everything in his power to gain muscle mass. He trained at least 5 days a week, he ate a healthy breakfast, lunch, and dinner along with a few snacks in between, and he even began to use a few scoops of whey protein every day. Yet after 2 years, not much had changed.

With his notable lack of success, his friends wondered why he kept this up, and even his parents confirmed that his dad had never been able to gain weight when he was John's age (insinuating that John wouldn't be able to, either). But just before John gave up all hope, an epiphany! At the time, a friend of his went away to a football training camp for a month and came back 15 pounds heavier. John was amazed. Probing him for his secrets, he told John that there weren't any secrets. Instead, at this camp, they were taught to eat five or six big meals per day. Angry, John told him that he already did that. But when he shared the actual meals with John, his jaw dropped. You see, when he said "big meals," John wasn't prepared for what he meant by "big." For example, take the size of the meal you have in your mind right now, and double it. Then double it again. Now we're talking about breakfast meals that consist of 12 whole eggs, four packets of plain instant oatmeal, and four slices of rye toast; lunches that consist of three whole-grain bagels, 1 pound of lean beef, and a huge salad; and dinners that consist of a full pound of pasta, a few cups of broccoli, and half a pound of lean ground beef. Not only did these guys eat these three big meals, but they would also eat and drink five whole grain bagels slathered with natural peanut butter and a liter of protein drink throughout the rest of the day.

Sound absurd? Well, not only does it sound absurd, it looked absurd. What a sight it is to behold such mass food consumption. However, eating this way made all the football-camp attendees bigger and stronger. And since it worked for them, John was definitely on board.

In the end, to make a long story short, utilizing these feeding techniques, John went from a 5'8", 150-pound guy (at 10 percent body fat) aspiring to bench press his own body weight to a 210-pound guy (at 12 percent body fat) bench-pressing 315 pounds for multiple reps. And all of this happened in just less than 2 years. Was John really hypertrophy-challenged, or was he simply an under-eater? We'll let you be the judge. But while you're pondering that question, it's time to move on to the next chapter, where we'll take a trip to the grocery store!

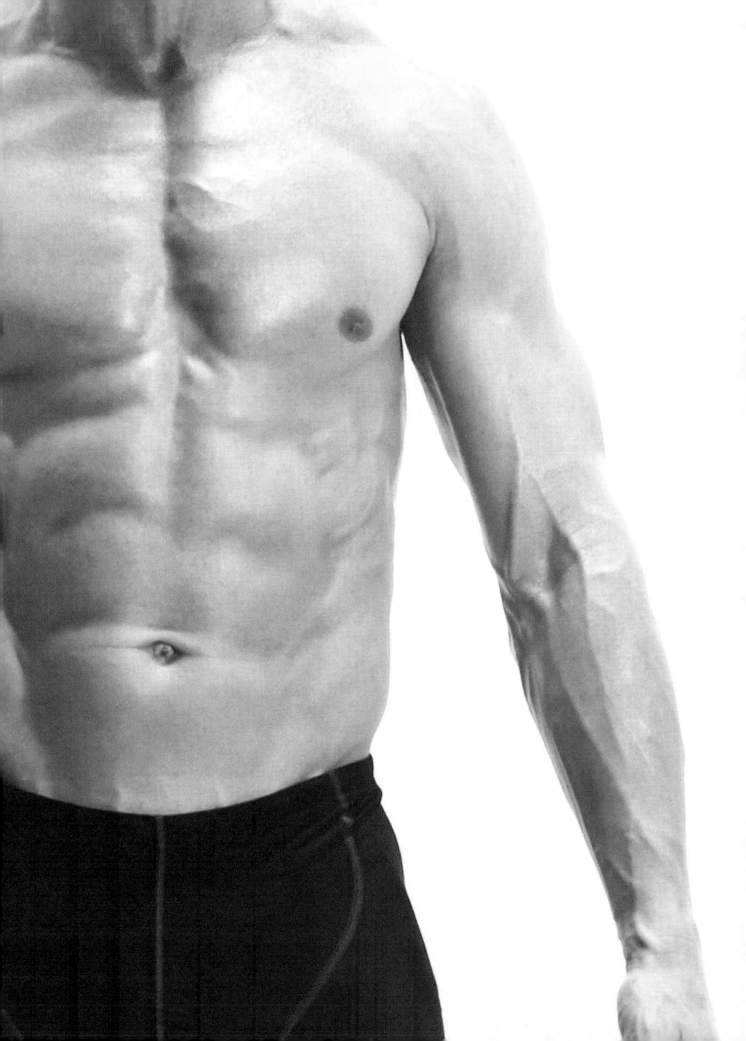

GO TO THE GROCERY STORE— NOW!

If you're interested in gaining muscle mass and have, in the past, either floundered ineffectually or simply failed to try, there are two ideas you're going to have to get comfortable with right away, so brace yourself.

Idea #1: To gain muscle mass, you're going to have to spend more money on groceries than you're currently spending (not necessarily a lot more, but more nonetheless).

Idea #2: To gain muscle mass, you're going to have to shop, cook, eat, and clean the kitchen more often than you're currently doing.

Sure, we're probably not supposed to tell you up front about the challenges you'll face, since most of the books out there nowadays seem to want to spin white lies, telling you how easy it is to get into great shape, how easy it is to lift weights, how easy it is to eat better. But the reality is this: It's only easy to do these things when you've prepared yourself mentally for the challenges that lie ahead and realize that it will take some time to accomplish your goals. You see, people typically overestimate how difficult things will be and underestimate how long they'll take. Expect to be able to gain weight or lose weight, for that matter, without seriously altering your current habits and taking the time to allow the new habits to sink in, and, of course, you'll fail. Truly, the old cliché "Insanity is doing the same thing over and over again and expecting a different result" has become a cliché for a reason; there's some truth to it.

Understanding that some of your habits have led to legs that only Colonel Sanders could love, you may be wondering what habits are in need of a change and what habits will direct you toward the path of muscle-building success? Well, we'll again be honest. We can't know exactly what your personal ineffective patterns are without sitting down with you in our clinic or chatting with you at www.scrawnytobrawny.com and assessing your current habits. However, in general, after working with thousands of clients, we do know that most people make some of the same mistakes with respect to muscle-building nutrition. Here are just a few:

Mistake #1: Eating Too Few Calories. Most people who want to get big simply eat too few calories. The body obeys the laws of thermodynamics (just a fancy physics word for describing how the body can't build muscle without extra energy around to build it with), and therefore, if you're losing weight, you're not taking enough energy in; if your weight is stable, you're balancing intake with output; if you're gaining weight, you're taking more energy in than you're burning. So if you're reading this book and want to get bigger, the solution should be relatively simple, right? No, don't eat the book! Pick up some food, and start eating it. By eating a greater number of calories than you're currently eating, you'll finally be able to put those high school physics lessons to good use. But rather than eating any old number of any old type of calories, you need to check out Chapter 13 for how much to eat and what to eat.

Mistake #2: Cupboards Are Bare. Most people live like Old Mother Hubbard. Ever have the experience of heading to the fridge to get something to eat and getting there to find nothing left that didn't have mold in it or on it? In order to ensure that you're getting enough food, you don't need a magic act; you need to ensure that your fridge and your cupboards are always stocked properly. And that's what we'll teach you how to do in this chapter.

Mistake #3: Failing to Plan Meals. Most people fail to eat enough calories because they fail to plan their meals. As you might imagine, another cliché works in nicely here. In nutrition, failing to plan is planning to fail. Trying to simply "eat on the go," "grab something on the way to work," or "catch a quick lunch with the guys from the mailroom" will serve only to accomplish one goal: to keep you looking average, just like everyone else. To transcend the typical physique, as you'll learn in Chapter 13, you should be eating about five or six meals per day (seven or eight meals counting your workout and post-workout drinks). So if you aren't sure what you're having for breakfast, for second breakfast, for lunch, for second lunch, for dinner, and for second dinner, chances are you'll make poor selections and/or skip meals altogether. Now that's a good recipe for success in your bid to win the World's *Weakest* Man title.

Mistake #4: Limited Food Choices. Most people eat only a limited range of foods each day. Because of convenience, social conditioning, food associations, etc., many people eat only a few foods each day, limiting the number of calories they're eating dramatically and limiting their vitamin and mineral intake. Think about it; list the different types of fruits and vegetables you ate yesterday. Seriously, take out a piece of paper, and write down the fruits and veggies you ate yesterday. We'll wait . . . So, did you eat the daily recommendation of six to eight servings of fruits and vegetables? Heck, did you meet that recommendation all of last week? If not, don't feel bad; very few of our clients do before they start working with us, and many of them are elite and professional athletes. The bottom line is this: If you're eating only a handful of different foods each day, you're limiting your muscle-building potential tremendously. In this chapter, we'll demonstrate the kind of variety it takes to succeed.

Mistake #5: Eating Infrequently. Most people eat only three "squares" a day. As you probably know, our societal feeding structure is centered on the three-meal day: breakfast, lunch, and dinner. What is this, prison? People—we're allowed to (and should) eat all day. Interestingly, when our society adopted this three-meal-a-day structure, no one thought to ask our physiology if this structure was best. As you might imagine, we're about to suggest that it's not best, especially if muscle gain is your goal. If you want to send those medium-size T-shirts to the Goodwill, once and for all, you'll have to eat when required, which means more often than most other "normal people." In Chapter 13, we'll outline exactly how often you should be eating.

Mistake #6: Mood Eating. Most people eat based on their mood and not on what their bodies need. We're sure you've seen these people in action. Do you know someone who overeats when "stressed out"? You probably do. But we're willing to bet you also know someone who doesn't eat at all when "stressed." So what's the difference between these two types of people? Only the fact that they've associated food with certain moods rather than treating food as sustenance, fuel for their engine. Think of it this way: You're about to take a long drive on a stretch of highway with no gas station. Do you fail to stop for gas before you hit the highway because you're "not in the mood"? Of course not. Think of eating in the same way. Eating fuels your metabolic engine. So it's time to *start* feeling like eating so that you can *stop* feeling like you're scrawny.

There you have it; we've laid out some of the common mistakes people make with respect to nutrition. Do any of these habits characterize your eating? If so, it's time to make the decision to get your habits working for you rather than against you. Regardless of whether you're currently a stress eater or a stress faster, a three-meals-a-day-only eater or a one-meal-a-day eater, or a wings-and-beer-when-out-with-the-boys eater, it's time to take an inventory of where you're falling short. The best way to do that is to think back to what you bought during your last trip to the grocery store, and compare your previous grocery list to the one we're about to present at the end of this chapter. After you've taken a mental note of the differences, we want you to then finish this chapter, close the book, and do what the title of the chapter says: Go to the Grocery Store—Now!

We're not kidding. Even if you've shopped already for the week (now you won't have to shop for 2 weeks). Even if you don't like any of the foods on this list (we'll teach you how to customize your list later on). Even if you have to take a taxi because someone stole your car (hope you had insurance). Even if you have to stand out front and beg for enough spare change to complete your purchase (get a job already!). We want you to go shopping and get used to the idea of making grocery shopping a planned event. In other words, we want you to eventually get to the point where you . . .

1. Shop at regular intervals, so you never run out of good, muscle-building nutrition. We suggest that many of our clients shop once per week. Since they're buying lots of fruits, vegetables, and meats, once per week is about right to ensure that nothing goes bad. Also, shopping once per week ensures that there are fewer

occasions in which they run out of food.

2. Visit the store with a planned list that'll cover you until the next shopping excursion. For now, take this book, and use the list on page 165 to shop from. Eventually, once you customize your intake, you'll need to make your own lists based on the number of calories you should be eating as well as which foods you're going to incorporate into your plan.

3. Spend only 15 to 20 minutes grocery shopping because you know exactly what you need and exactly where it's located. Using this system, there's no walking up and down the aisles, wasting time, being tempted by the newest barbecue sauce or frozen entrée. In this system, shopping becomes a targeted event, and you're in and out of the store in a flash.

4. Avoid all the aisles that contain foods not conducive to your goals. Most often, much of the best food is found around the perimeter of the grocery store. Around the perimeter, you'll find the produce section (fruits, vegetables, potatoes, nuts, etc.), the meat section (chicken, lean beef, fish, etc.), the bakery section (choose the fresh whole-grain breads and not the desserts, please), and the dairy aisle (cottage cheese, plain yogurt, eggs, etc.). Sure, the middle aisles might have to be visited from time to time. But be on guard; it's the aisles in the middle (snacks, juices, etc.) that can get you into trouble with their pretty packaging and "magically delicious" flavors. Stay away from the bright, shiny objects.

So as you can see, we've got this gettin'-big shopping system down to a science. But why all the rules? Well, if you're looking in the mirror and aren't liking what you see, chances are you've got your own set of rules, and these rules are perfect for creating a sorry physique. Our rules are perfect for creating a perfect physique. So which would you like to follow again? In all seriousness, when you're trying to repattern your life, there's little room for winging it. Although training to gain muscle mass is fun, eating to gain muscle mass is fun, and watching other people's faces as they appreciate your new muscle mass is fun, exchanging old, ineffectual habits for new habits isn't always fun; it can be difficult. However, like all good investments, the larger the amount of capital you're willing to put into the investment, the larger the reward.

It's time for you to do yourself a favor. Take this book to the grocery store with you *right now*, and buy the groceries listed on the opposite page. Then, when you come back with your culinary bounty, move on to the next chapter. In it, we'll teach you how to make what we call the "First Supper."

Grocery shopping, muscle-building-style, is definitely an art. If you've not yet mastered the art, here are a few tips for navigating the many selections in your store.

Fruit and vegetable tips

1. Make it simple on yourself, and pick up fresh fruits and vegetables that are packaged and prepared in a way closest to how you'll eat them.

GROCERY LIST

- 7 large bags fresh spinach
- 3 large bags fresh carrots
- 2 pineapples, either fresh or precut
- 7 apples
- 7 plums (or oranges, pears, etc.)
- 4 bananas
- 7 potatoes/yams
- 1 bag of quinoa (ancient grain)
- 1 lemon
- 1 clove garlic
- 4 large red bell peppers
- 1 onion
- 1 pound walnuts

- 1 container nonstick cooking spray
- 1 box high-fiber cereal
- 1 jar pesto
- 1 box green tea
- 1 container apple cider vinegar
- 1 bottle flax oil
- 1 bottle extra virgin olive oil
- 7 pounds extra lean ground beef
- 3 packages chicken or turkey sausage

- 7 containers egg whites
- 1 dozen omega-3 eggs
- 1/2 pound sliced cheese
- 2 large containers plain yogurt
- 2-pound container whey protein
- 1 container carbohydrate/sports drink
- 1 bottle salmon oil/fish oil capsules

For example, pick up prewashed, bagged spinach leaves; precut pineapple; baby carrots, etc. These selections will ensure that making your meals is a much less time-consuming endeavor for you or whatever sucker you rope into cooking for you.

2. Don't buy canned fruits and vegetables. They've got all kinds of nasty stuff you don't want going into your body (for you science savvy, that's another way of saying they contain bisphenol A and some other potential carcinogens).

3. Although organic produce may contain a higher vitamin and mineral count as well as fewer pesticides, the most important thing is for you to simply get more fruits and vegetables in your diet. So buy the best vegetables you can afford, focusing on

getting the entire recommended amount. If you can easily find and afford organics or pesticide-free foods, great. If not, pick up what you can; just be sure it's not actually *in* a can.

Oils, vinegars, sprays, grains, and teas

1. Just like with the veggies, organic is probably best. However, if you can't find organic, or it's too expensive, adding the "regular" brands will still do wonders for your physique.

2. Most of these products can be found in the same section of your grocery store (the natural foods section). The quinoa (pronounced KEEN-wah) is usually also found in this section. If your store doesn't have such a section, you'll have to venture into the perilous

165

"aisles" to find your teas, oils, and ancient grains.

3. As far as cereal, simply pick up a high-fiber cereal that you enjoy. Cereals coated with sugar or full of marshmallow playthings don't count.

Meats

1. Just as with the other products, organic meats may be best. However, don't let the lack of organic meat availability (this stuff is hard to find) stand in your way. If you insist on organics, you may have to visit your local butcher and have him point you in the right direction.

2. To ensure the freshest cuts, simply make friends with your local butcher or the butcher at your local grocery store. But don't start off by telling him that you "love their meat." Mike did that once and was banned from the store for life. If you get to know the butcher, he'll be able to tell you which days to find the freshest cuts. Pick up your beef and chicken on those days to ensure better shelf life.

3. When buying red meat, be sure to pick up ground beef that's extra lean. Some stores will refer to it as "extra lean," others as "93 percent lean," others as "ground sirloin." When buying chicken breast, be sure to pick up skinless, boneless chicken breast. Sure, the price per pound is higher. But if you get the cheaper stuff, you'll be paying for the junk (bones and skin) that you'll be throwing away anyway. Unless you're a Viking and prefer to

gnaw on the bones. And seek out turkey or chicken sausage. This stuff tastes great!

Eggs and dairy

1. In your dairy section, you'll easily be able to find egg whites in cartons. When these things first appeared on the market, a collective sigh of relief could be heard from weightlifters everywhere. No more cracking and separating, these cartons can simply be poured out into a pan (sprayed with your nonstick cooking spray from above) and scrambled or made into an omelet.

2. With respect to yogurt, another thing to remember is that fruity yogurts are to be left on the shelves. These products have much less protein and much more sugar. Instead, pick up some regular (not fat-reduced), plain yogurt. Balkan style is especially good, but you don't need to find the fancy stuff. Rather, the economy tub of plain yogurt is perfect.

Supplements

1. Some grocery stores actually have small supplement sections in them. If this is the case in your store, this is where you can pick up your fish oil, protein supplements, and powdered sports drink. If not, you'll have to find a local supplement store for your supplements.

2. As indicated, you'll be picking up some whey protein powder and some sports drink powder. Both of these are relatively inexpensive. When selecting whey protein, to ensure you're not getting a whole bunch of lactose or other potential allergens, pick up some CFM whey isolates (ask the salesperson to direct you to this type of whey protein). When selecting a sports drink powder, simply pick a powder that contains simple carbohydrate and no other fancy bells and whistles. We'll go into detail on supplements in Chapter 16.

3. Your final supplement purchase will be fish oil. Simply look for "salmon oil" or "fish oil" (cod liver oil *will not* do). To ensure you've found the right stuff, look at the back of the label, and add up the amount of EPA and DHA per serving. If the total adds up to anywhere from 300 to 600 mg per serving, jump up and down; you've got a winner.

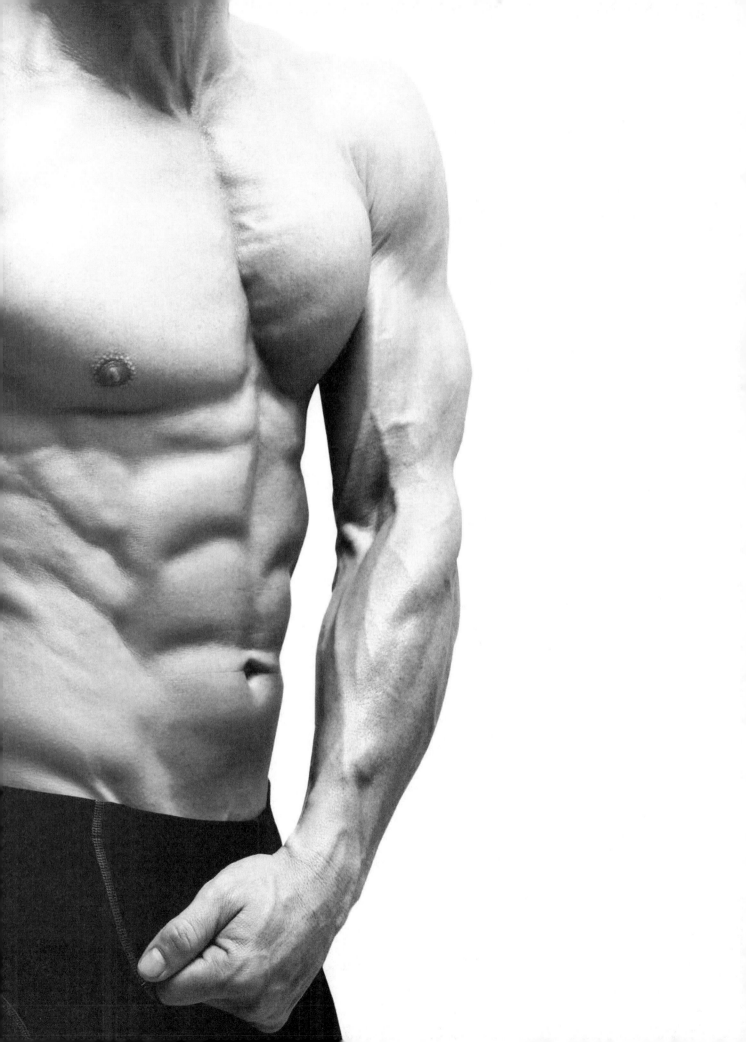

MAKING THE FIRST SUPPER

Been to the grocery store? If not, we strongly recommend that you *stop reading*, and start shopping. Yeah, we know, we're stubborn. But you see, although this book is educational, it's not an academic book. It's not designed expressly to fill your head with facts, knowledge, and/or trivia. It's designed to get you to take action today. Remember the old adage: "Knowledge is power"? Well that's not true. Knowledge isn't power; knowledge is information. Power comes from *applied* knowledge. And applied knowledge is action.

Although we'll dive into nutrition program design later in the book, showing you exactly what you should be eating day in and day out and exactly how to put together a nutrition program from start to finish, right now, we want to introduce you to the concept of the "First Supper." We call your next meal the First Supper because it, quite simply, represents your initiation into the world of the wide. So why the fancy name, why the pomp and circumstance? Well, this first meal should represent more than a feeding opportunity for you. It should represent the beginning of your new habits, the beginning of your new nutritional program, the beginning of a whole lot of hard work culminating in a whole lot of muscle mass.

Ever hear the old saying: Today is the first day of the rest of your life? Well, you can think of the First Supper as the first meal of the rest of your diet. If you plan on really taking a serious run at this gettin' big thing, this is your first milestone in your quest for serious muscle. Think about it this way: Up until now, you haven't been doing what it takes to get bigger (if you had, then you wouldn't be reading this book). So before this meal, you've been eating like a scrawny guy. But after this meal, everything will have changed. After this meal, you'll be eating like the big boys. And here's how it's done.

The First Supper Ingredients

8 ounces (225 grams) extra lean ground beef

1 omega-3 egg

1 tablespoon pesto

Chopped onion and pepper

4 ounces (110 grams) spinach

4 ounces (110 grams) carrots

1 tablespoon walnuts

1 apple, chopped

1 tablespoon flax oil

2 tablespoons apple cider vinegar

1 slice cheese

)) Preparing the meat

1. Throw the beef, egg, pesto, and a small amount of chopped onion and pepper in a bowl.

2. With these ingredients, form 1 large burger patty (gettin' those hands dirty, of course).

3. If you have a grill (outdoor or indoor), you can slap it on the grill. If not, you can either place it in a pan (sprayed with the cooking spray you bought and sitting on medium heat), or place it in the oven at 400 degrees.

)) Preparing the vegetables

1. While the burger is cooking, place the spinach, carrots, walnuts, and apple in a bowl.

2. Sprinkle the flax oil and apple cider vinegar on top.

)) Finishing the meal

1. Once the burger is done cooking, add the cheese to the top.

2. Serve the burger, salad, and 500 milliliters of water.

So that's the First Supper. Now that you've read about it, it's time to go cook it. Make sure you do that right away. And after having done so, you can read on.

Okay, now that you've eaten the First Supper, it's time to learn something about it. The meal you just ate provided you with 810 calories, 62 grams of protein, 39 grams of low glycemic index carbohydrate (about 10 grams of fiber), and 48 grams of fat (one-third of the fat coming from saturated fatty acids, one-third from monounsaturated fatty acids, and one-third from polyunsaturated fatty acids). Not only that, the meal was packed with micronu-

trients like B-vitamins, iron, calcium, etc. Pat yourself on the back because you just ate healthier in one meal than some North Americans eat all day and others all week!

In terms of the meal composition, we refer to this meal as a protein plus fat meal (P + F). We call it this because 30 percent of the calories in this meal come from protein and 52 percent come from fat. Later in the book, we'll discuss this distinction in greater detail. However, for now, trust us when we say that P + F meals are optimal during specific times of the day while protein plus carbohydrate (P + C) meals are optimal during other times. Interested in what a P + C meal would look like? Here's an example:

P + C Meal Ingredients

1/2 cup quinoa

8 ounces (225 grams) extra lean ground beef

1 egg white

2 tablespoons fresh garlic

Chopped onion and pepper

4 ounces (110 grams) spinach

4 ounces (110 grams) carrots

1 apple, chopped

2 tablespoons apple cider vinegar

3 fish oil capsules

)) Preparing the quinoa

1. Bring 1 1/2 cups of water to a boil.

2. Prepare meat and vegetables while waiting for it to boil.

3. Add quinoa to the water, and stir periodically until water evaporates.

4. Place in a bowl.

)) Preparing the meat

1. With your hands, mix the beef, egg white, garlic, and a small amount of chopped onion and pepper in a bowl.

2. Place the ingredients into a pan (sprayed with the cooking spray you bought and sitting on medium heat) and cook, continually breaking up the meat, so it stays ground.

3. When the quinoa is ready, stir the cooked meat into it.

» Preparing the vegetables

1. While the meat is cooking, place the spinach, carrots, and apple in a bowl.

2. Sprinkle the vinegar on top.

» Finishing the meal

Serve the meal with 3 fish oil capsules and 500 milliliters of water.

Like the P + F meal, this one contains about 800 calories. However, the macronutrient content differs. In this meal, 31 percent of the calories in this meal come from protein and 50 percent from carbohydrate (with only 19 percent from fat). You can now see why this meal is obviously called a protein plus carbohydrate meal (P + C).

Now that you've been exposed to P + F and P + C meals, we have to emphasize a point we made in the nutrition introduction. Again, most people, based on their own past experiences, have some internal notion of how much food should be enough, how many calories they should try to eat, and how much protein, carbohydrate, and fat is enough or too much. For example, whether you feel this way or not, I know there are a number of fat phobics out there objecting to the amount of fat in our P + F meal: "48 grams of fat in one meal; isn't that too much?" Interestingly, though, while there are some afraid of the fat, there are others, carb phobics, accepting these fat numbers but objecting to the carbohydrate content: "100 grams of carbs in one meal; isn't that too much?" And while some aren't concerned with the fat or carbohydrate content, there are protein phobics worried about the protein content: "64 grams of protein in one meal; isn't that too much?" How do we address these objections?

We don't. After all, one of us has a PhD with a focus in exercise nutrition. If we're not making these objections, they're probably not valid. You see, most of these types of objections aren't based in physiological reality. They are based on erroneous notions of how food and calories are metabolized.

The best we can do right now is tell you to trust us. Don't second-guess the program. Just follow it, and decide whether it's good or not after you've recorded your results, not before. Again, this game is an *outcome-based* one. Remember the Science Link (John's company) tag line: "No matter how beautiful the strategy, you should occasionally look at the results."

And if our previous paragraph wasn't enough to convince you to overcome your macronutrient phobias, here's another way of thinking about the problem. In Chapter 13, we'll teach you how to calculate your total energy needs for the day. Since your total energy intake (calories) is the most important determinant of whether you'll gain weight, lose weight, or stay the same, this is a critical component of designing your nutritional program.

Since we haven't figured out your numbers yet, let's go through an example. Since many of the hypertrophy-challenged have screaming metabolisms, a 6'1", 190-pound ectomorph may need in the neighborhood of 4,000 to 5,000 calories per day if he hopes to gain muscle. If that's you, tell your secretary to cancel all appointments; you're going to be spending the day eating! Breaking these 4,000 to 5,000 calories down, that comes to six to eight meals of about 600 to 800 calories each. Now, pray tell, how are you supposed to get all 600 to 800 calories multiple times per day without taking in a large number of proteins, carbs, and fats? The easy answer: There's no way.

Okay, now that we've eaten the First Supper, and you've been initiated, it's time to find your way to the next milestone on the road toward muscledom. Now that you've gotten an acute taste of what it takes to eat for big muscles and good health, it's time to figure out how to tailor these meals to your specific, individual needs. That's right, in Chapter 13, we're going to teach you how.

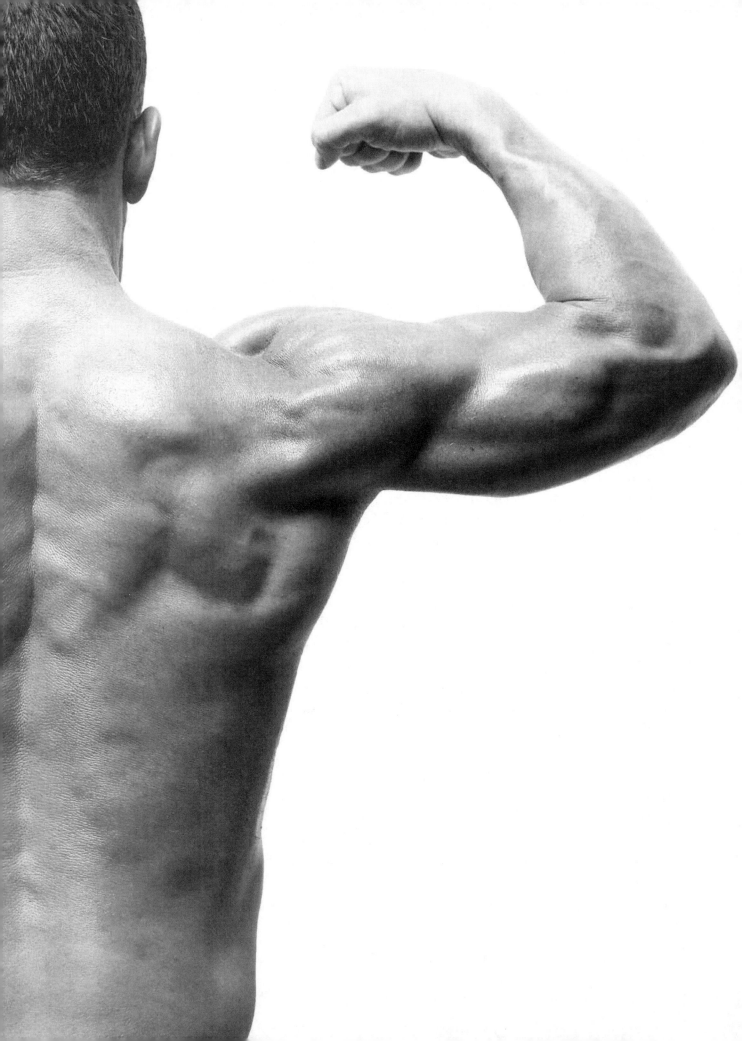

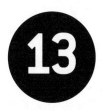

GETTING BIGGER IS A BATTLE— YOUR WEAPON IS A FORK

》》As discussed earlier, increased muscle mass comes as a direct result of creating a muscle-producing environment. Of course, this means you need to train hard. But training hard alone is never enough. You see, measurable increases in muscle mass come as a direct result of stimulating the muscle to build (in the gym) and then providing the muscle with raw materials to do the building (in the kitchen). You can think of it this way: By hitting the gym, you're hiring a bunch of skilled bricklayers to build your house. Without bricks, however, these bricklayers have nothing to do but sit around, shouting catcalls at any females walking by. But give these guys some bricks, and although they'll still probably shout catcalls, they'll build the house. So you see; it's that environment thing again. Question: How effectively can bricklayers work in a brickless environment? If you answered: about as effectively as you can build muscle in a low-calorie, poor-nutrient environment, you're catching on.

You simply must get comfortable with the idea that although exercise itself offers a number of inherent health benefits, this book's all about gaining muscle. And building muscle comes from training hard and eating lots of groceries. In the previous chapters, we sent you to the grocery store and encouraged you to start your assault on the world of the wide. Assuming you followed through, stocked the fridge, and made The First Supper, it's time to plan out the rest of your nutrition program, starting with your energy/calorie needs.

DETERMINING ENERGY/CALORIE NEEDS

In the past, you've probably heard experts offer very simple multipliers to determine energy needs. These experts might tell you to multiply your body mass by 20 to determine how many kcal (kilocalories) per day you need to eat. For example, if you are 200 pounds, you need to eat 200 × 20 kcal, or 4,000 kcal. While these strategies are pretty basic and simple to apply, they don't take into account your personal lifestyle, training habits, etc. To remedy this, we're going to use a formula that's a bit more complex. While it lacks simplicity, our formula offers a much more detailed and individualized approach that can be tweaked based on your daily activity levels and training schedule. At this point, you'll need some paper, a writing utensil, and a calculator. Once you've got these, it's time to figure out how much food you'll need to eat.

Step #1: Resting Metabolic Rate

Resting metabolic rate, or RMR, is the amount of energy your body needs to maintain physiological functioning without movement. The RMR is usually measured while lying quietly since that represents the most inactive part of your day. Now, although it might not subjectively "feel" like you're expending a lot of energy while lying in bed in the morning, about 50 to 70 percent of your total daily energy expenditure (depending on how active you are) comes from the constant energy cost of RMR. Therefore, if you stayed in bed all day, your energy needs would probably drop by only about 40 percent. Since RMR represents only the amount of energy needed to be alive (with minimal activity), it obviously doesn't include the cost of getting your butt out of bed, brushing your teeth, or hitting the gym. So after we determine RMR, we'll calculate those activity numbers and add them in.

But first, let's calculate RMR. The following predictive RMR equation is taken from a study published in 1999 by A. DeLorenzo and colleagues at the University of Rome. These scientists directly measured the RMR of a group of 51 male athletes and determined that this equation (known as the Cunningham equation) predicted the RMR to within 59 kcal. In addition to the men studied in the DeLorenzo study, the Cunningham equation has also been validated in female athletes. In 1996, J. Thompson and colleagues at the University of North Carolina measured the RMR of 24 athletic men and 13 athletic women and determined that the Cunningham equation was accurate to within 158 kcal for men and 103 kcal for women. These studies clearly show that the Cunningham equation is accurate for use in athletic populations who exercise regularly.

CALCULATING RMR—
THE CUNNINGHAM EQUATION

To start off with, you need to take your body mass in pounds and convert it to kilograms. (International readers, please bear with us silly nonmetric Americans for a moment.) This is a simple conversion. Just divide your body weight by 2.2 to get your mass in kilograms. For example, a 200-pound man would be 200 ÷ 2.2 or 90.91 kg.

Next take your percent fat (see "Methods of Determining Body Fat" on page 176 for how to determine your percent fat), and multiply it by your body mass (which is now in kilograms). This will give you your fat mass (FM) in kilograms. For example, a 90.91-kg man at 5 percent fat would have 90.91 × 0.05 or 4.55 kg of fat. If you're not writing this down, you'd better!

Next, simply subtract this last number from your total weight in kilograms, and you'll have your fat-free mass (FFM) in kilograms. For example, a 90.91-kg man with 4.55 kg of fat would have 90.91 − 4.55 or 86.36 kg of FFM.

Now that we've determined that our individual has 86.36 kg of FFM, we can plug this number into the Cunningham Formula as follows:

RMR = 500 + [22 × fat-free mass (in kilograms)]

RMR = 500 + [22 × 86.36]

RMR = 500 + 1,899.92

RMR = 2,399.92 kcal

Remember, of course, that these numbers are for a hypothetical trainee who is 200 pounds and 5 percent body fat. To figure out your own numbers, repeat the process, plugging in your own body mass and body-fat numbers.

Step #2: Thermic Effect of Food

The Thermic Effect of Food, or TEF, represents the heat produced as a direct function of eating. In other words, it's the number of kilocalories required to digest, absorb, and metabolize your ingested food intake. The TEF typically represents about 10 to 15 percent of your total daily energy expenditure. Different macronutrients elicit a different thermic response. Protein [>] carbohydrate [>] fat.

DETERMINING THE THERMIC EFFECT OF FOOD

To determine the TEF, you need to multiply your original RMR value by 0.10 for a moderate-protein diet or 0.15 for a high-protein diet. Since you'll be following our program, and this program requires a relatively high-protein diet, multiply your RMR by 0.15. Keeping with our example of a 200-pound individual with 5 percent body fat:

TEF = RMR × 0.15

TEF = 2,399.92 × 0.15

TEF = 359.99

Now, in adding TEF to RMR, our model individual has a new energy requirement of 2,399.92 + 359.99 or 2,759.90 kcal. Now do the same for your own numbers.

Step #3: Activity Thermogenesis

Activity Thermogenesis represents the amount of energy your body uses during all activity. This means how many calories you need to move your butt around during the day, including walking out to your car in the morning, scraping the ice off the damn thing in the winter, driving to work, sitting at your desk, going to the coffee machine, going to lunch with the boss, and of course, training after work. Now, activity thermogenesis can be divided into two components: nonexercise activity thermogenesis (NEAT) and exercise-related activity thermogenesis (ERAT). In all, activity thermogenesis can make up anywhere from 15 to 50 percent of your total daily energy expenditure based on how active you are.

NONEXERCISE ACTIVITY THERMOGENESIS

At this point we want to correct your daily RMR number by adding your NEAT to it. To do so, we'll multiply the original RMR, calculated above, by an activity factor (representing NEAT) that fits your daily routine. According to J. Levine, renowned researcher at the Mayo Clinic, the following represent accurate multipliers for the determination of total daily energy expenditure:

1.2 to 1.3 for bed- or chair-ridden individuals

1.4 to 1.5 for sedentary occupation without daily movement

1.5 to 1.6 for sedentary occupation with daily movement

1.6 to 1.7 for occupation with prolonged standing

1.9 to 2.1 for strenuous work or high leisure activity

Note: Don't consider your daily workout when choosing a number. Just choose your nonexercise activity. For example, assuming our 200-pound individual with 5 percent fat works in an office and sits at a desk for most of the day, he would choose 1.45 as his NEAT multiplier.

RMR + NEAT = RMR × NEAT factor

RMR + NEAT = 2,399.92 × 1.45

RMR + NEAT = 3,479.88 kcal

At this point, by adding your TEF number to your RMR + NEAT number, you'll have your RMR + NEAT + TEF. This number represents your total daily energy expenditure on nonworkout days. For our example above:

RMR + NEAT + TEF = 3,479.88 + 359.98

RMR + NEAT + TEF = 3,839.86

Again, this last number 3,839.86 kcal represents total daily energy expenditure on nonworkout days for our example individual above. Now do the same for your own numbers; determine which multiplier you need to use, and calculate your RMR + NEAT. Then add in your TEF, and you've got your energy needs for nonworkout days.

DETERMINING EXERCISE-RELATED ACTIVITY THERMOGENESIS

Moving right along to the next set of calculations, we need to determine how much energy

METHODS OF DETERMINING BODY FAT

The measurement of body fat or body composition is a hotly debated topic. The reason is that it's impossible to measure your actual body-fat percentage without blending your body up and doing a chemical digest of the remains. Since that would definitely hurt your progress in the gym, indirect measures of body composition assessment have been created to attempt to predict body composition. Between these methods, there is considerable variability. Therefore, if you get tested in one gym by the "pinch method" and in another gym on one of those fancy impedance scales, your body fat percentage could be as much as 10 percent different. If you're following our program and are measured today at 10 percent fat and then next week at 20 percent fat, we're sure you won't buy any of our future books. So, in an attempt to preserve future sales, we hope to give you some tips below for measuring body composition.

When trying to determine your body-fat percentage, there are three important criteria for ensuring a good test. The first is accuracy; does the test give you a reasonably accurate result? The second is reliability; if you were to do 10 tests in a row, would the results come out similarly? And the third is convenience; can you routinely have this test performed?

Using these three criteria, we rate several of the main body composition assessment methods below.

1. Body mass index. Some facilities use body mass index, determined by weight (in kg) ÷ height squared (in cm), as an index of body composition. Although this method is easy, since it determines only the relationship between height and weight with no regard for the composition of that weight, the Body Mass Index does not provide an accurate assessment of body composition.

2. Skinfold testing. Skinfold testing requires the use of a special caliper that measures the thickness (in millimeters) of pinched skin at several body locations. These measurements are then plugged into an equation to predict body-fat percentage. This method of testing is easy to perform and, if done *consistently by the same qualified professional,* is both accurate and reliable. In addition, this measurement tool allows for the measurement of skin thickness at several locations, allowing you to monitor fat loss in specific areas. In our estimation, a seven-site skinfold test is optimal for monitoring overall body-fat percentage and site-specific fat loss. When it's time to get your body composition tested, contact your local gym or the exercise you'll need on training days by figuring out your exercise-related activity thermogenesis. This can be simply by multiplying your total body mass in kilograms (as calculated above) by the duration of your exercise (in hours) and again multiplied by the MET value of the exercise you are performing. So what's a MET? No, not an overpaid, under-achieving ballplayer from New York. It's a metabolic equivalency unit or metabolic multiplier. One MET is equal to your resting metabolic rate while 10 METs is equal to 10× your resting metabolic rate. So here's the formula and a sample calculation based on our 200-pound individual with 5 percent fat. Let's assume that on training days, he exercises for 90 minutes, and his exercise is heavy weight training.

ERAT = Body Mass (kg) × Duration (hours) × MET

ERAT = 90.91 kg × 1.5 hr × 6 METS

ERAT = 818.19 kcal

This calculation demonstrates that our example lifter expends 818.19 calories during training. Add this number (818.19 kcal) to the number determined above for nonworkout days (3,839.64 kcal),

program at your local university, and begin a relationship with one individual who is qualified to take these measurements. Since you'll want these taken regularly and properly, this is a wise investment. Again, ensure that this individual will always be the person taking your measurements, and make sure they keep a record of your overall fat percentage and your seven individual skinfolds.

3. Bioelectric impedance. This method requires a handheld device or a scale-type device to send an imperceptible electric current through your body. The rate at which this current travels through and back out of your body is measured, and this rate is directly related to your overall body water content (about 70 percent of your body mass is water). Since body water is directly related to body-fat percentage, your machine will do a quick calculation to predict your body fat. This method of body-fat prediction, while very easy, is known to present accuracy problems. If it says you're 20 percent fat, you could be anywhere from 15 to 25 percent. That's too big a margin for our liking, especially since you'll be using it in this chapter to predict your energy needs. Fortunately, the reliability of this method is not too

bad. If it's all you have access to, for a ballpark figure, it's better than nothing for tracking your progress.

4. Displacement methods. Hydrostatic or underwater weighing and the Bod Pod are two displacement methods of determining body composition. Hydrostatic testing provides a measure of water displacement, while the Bod Pod provides a measure of air displacement. Since your body volume is directly proportional to the amount of water or air you displace when placed in a chamber of water or air, and your body volume is directly proportional to your body fat, these methods provide a good measure of body composition. While these methods are both accurate and reliable, it's often difficult to find a facility that offers them, and if you do, it tends to be more expensive to have these tests performed. Even though these methods might be a bit better than skinfold methods, we still recommend skinfold testing unless you have access to a laboratory in which you can be regularly measured.

In the end, when trying to determine your body composition, the best advice we can give you is to pick one method, stick with it, and get tested regularly. This is the only way to effectively track your progress with any degree of certainty.

GETTING BIGGER IS A BATTLE—YOUR WEAPON IS A FORK

and you've got a total energy demand of 4,657.83 kcal on training days.

A quick review of our calculations done on our 200-pound individual with 5 percent body fat demonstrates that the main components of total daily energy expenditure are RMR, NEAT, TEF, and ERAT. Again, to derive these for yourself, you need to complete these steps:

1. Determine RMR (RMR = 500 + [22 × FFM])

2. Determine TEF (TEF = RMR × 0.15)

3. Determine RMR + NEAT (RMR + NEAT = RMR × NEAT factor)

4. Determine RMR + NEAT + TEF (add TEF to #3)

5. Determine ERAT (ERAT = Mass (kg) × Duration (hr) × MET)

6. Determine total daily energy expenditure (add ERAT to calculated RMR + NEAT + TEF)

In following the steps above, we see that our example lifter needs about 3,800 kcal on nontraining days and about 4,600 kcal on training days. Seem like a lot of food? You bet it does! For a complete breakdown of how much food it takes to ingest 4,000 kcal, see the meals on the opposite page.

With this big list of meals, it should now be clear to you why we keep saying that many individuals who think they're muscularly challenged are simply hungry mesomorphs, waiting for enough food to grow! Simply put, they have little idea of just how much food they must eat and therefore fall miserably short. As we said earlier, we don't like the term hardgainer. One of the reasons is that the only thing the average hardgainer seems to be hard of is hearing. No matter how many times we say that they need to eat more, they never seem to listen. Remember, getting big is a battle, and your weapon is a fork. If you're not growing, it's because you're not using that fork judiciously enough.

BUT I CAN'T IMAGINE EATING THIS MUCH FOOD

While the nutritional system outlined in this book has been well validated in a population of thousands of clients, it's constantly brought to our attention that this is a lot of food, and the average person can't image eating this much food in a day, let alone actually getting through a week or a month of eating like this. Of course, we appreciate this objection. But in all honesty, this is the same objection that keeps people average in every walk of life. Those individuals who "can't imagine" working weekends won't advance in their profession. Those athletes who "can't imagine" training 6 to 8 hours per day won't become world class. Those entrepreneurs who "can't imagine" risking

MET VALUES FOR COMMON ACTIVITIES

High-impact aerobics	7	High-intensity running	18
Low-impact aerobics	5	Low-intensity running	7
High-intensity cycling	12	Circuit-type training	8
Low-intensity cycling	3	Intense free-weight lifting	6
High-intensity walking	6.5	Moderate machine training	3
Low-intensity walking	2.5		

4,600-KCAL MENU FOR THE HYPERTROPHY-CHALLENGED

MEAL #1

12 egg whites

1 slice regular cheese

Chopped fresh veggies

1 tablespoon flax oil

2 fish oil capsules

1 cup green tea

MEAL #2

1 cup organic yogurt

1 scoop protein powder

2 fish oil capsules

MEAL #3

2 chicken sausage links

Organic spinach

1 cup organic carrots

2 tablespoons apple-cider vinegar

1 tablespoon flax oil

4 fish oil capsules

MEAL #4 PRE-WORKOUT

1 serving recovery drink

MEAL #5 DURING WORKOUT

1 serving recovery drink

MEAL #6 IMMEDIATELY AFTER WORKOUT

1 serving recovery drink

MEAL #7

1 cup yogurt

1 scoop protein powder

1 or 2 pieces fruit

2½ cups cereal

MEAL #8

4 oz. lean beef

Organic spinach

1 cup organic carrots

2 tablespoons apple-cider vinegar

½ cup quinoa (or yam)

1 piece fruit

MEAL #9

4 oz. lean beef

Organic spinach

1 cup organic carrots

2 tablespoons apple-cider vinegar

1 tablespoon olive oil

2 fish oil capsules

¼ cup cashews

large financial losses with a big investment will never become financially independent.

The nutritional system outlined in this book is an honest, proven, and scientific process that will definitely help you achieve your express goal—to gain muscle mass the natural way. There are hundreds of ways to fail. This book presents the way to succeed. Therefore, as we tell our clients in person, our job is not to make it easier for you. Our job is to tell you exactly what it'll take to achieve what seems to be a difficult goal. We also want to reiterate that difficult goals are achievable. However, they are achievable only when you know exactly what it takes to accomplish them. This book tells you what it takes. Do less than we tell you to do, and you'll achieve less than what we promise you can expect.

Now don't get us wrong and adopt an "all or none" approach. Just because some readers may choose not to follow *all* the principles discussed here, that doesn't mean that the system is doomed to failure, and they should abandon a sinking ship. After all, training hard and making better nutritional choices will definitely improve their bodies and help them get more muscular.

But in this specific case, if you truly want to go from Scrawny to Brawny, you're going to have to break out of the "comfort zone" that dictates what's normal and take the necessary steps toward improvement. The Scrawny to Brawny project is about making significant changes to your body. Significant changes *are not* achieved through using the same mindset you currently employ. Significant changes require an overhaul. In buying this book, you made a decision to learn how to build big muscles that get you noticed. In following our system, you're making a decision to do what it takes to get those muscles. There are no shortcuts.

SAME FORMULAS
FOR EVERYONE?

While we've just gone through the lengthy process of evaluating your calorie needs, it's time for us to make the clear picture presented above a bit blurry. It's time to discuss the idea of individual differences with respect to metabolic rate. Despite being able to calculate individual energy expenditure components as we've done above, customizing these calorie calculations always requires a bit of fine-tuning. You see, the calculations above work very well for the average trainee. However, with any population sample (in other words, with every group of people), there are people above the average and below. Therefore, some trainees may need more calories than this formula suggests and others fewer calories. I know what you're thinking: Doesn't this invalidate our calculations? Not really. The calculations bring us very close to what you need to be eating, and without a visit to our clinic or Web site, they're as close as you'll get from a book. So start with the calculations above, and then, after a bit of fine-tuning (as described below), you can become the designer of your own perfect plan.

Before delving into the specific adjustments you might need to make, however, we're going to begin with a quick discussion of why these individual differences are present in the first place and list some signs that indicate that you might respond differently than the average trainee.

It should be no surprise that some people can seemingly eat and eat yet not gain weight. Since you're reading this book, you may be one of them. That's right, if your friends constantly ask, "where you put it all" or "if you have a tapeworm" or "if you've got a hollow leg," chances are you're definitely one of them. But while some people can eat and eat without gaining weight, I'm sure you know more than a handful of individuals who don't eat very much or very often yet seem to easily pack on the pounds. These are the people who claim to "just gain weight by looking at food" (although I've never really figured out how that exactly worked).

So what's the deal? How can we have such different responses to feeding? Well, for starters, it's very difficult to make comparisons because people's *perceptions* of what they eat and what they *really* eat are often worlds apart. There are anorexic women out there who eat less than 1,000 kcal per day and still think they eat "like a pig." And there are obese individuals out there who eat "like birds" only to find out that they're taking in 3,000 kcal per day. So again, perceptions aren't always accurate. But mistaken perceptions aside, there is a good bit of scientific evidence showing that when energy intake is well controlled, some people seem to be more prone to weight gain than others. Likewise, others seem to be more weight-gain resistant than others.

To demonstrate this phenomenon, a landmark study appeared in *Science* in 1999, authored by James Levine, M.D., and colleagues from the Mayo Clinic. This study was designed to measure the effects of controlled overeating on weight gain. In the study, the researchers fed 16 nonobese subjects an extra 1,000 kcal per day above their measured maintenance kilocalorie needs for a total of 8 weeks. That's an extra 56,000 to 60,000 kcal over 2 months. If all those kilocalories were converted directly into fat, that would amount to about 16 to 17 pounds of blubber. Interestingly, while the average fat gain was 2.83 kg (or 6.23 pounds), there was a huge, tenfold variation in the amount of fat gained between subjects. Some of the subjects gained less than 0.50 kg (1.10 pound) of fat. We'll call these individuals fat-gain resistant. And some of them gained more than 4.00 kg (8.80 pounds) of fat. We'll call these individuals fat-gain prone. Considering the fact that all subjects were overfed to the same magnitude, these data provide a huge clue about why some people might be able to eat much,

much more than others without putting on weight.

Now we suspect that many of you hypertrophy-challenged individuals out there (including you ectomorphs) have some degree of weight-gain resistance, just like a number of the subjects in the study above. What gives us this idea? Well, in a study published by Christoph Raschka [*Schweiz Z Sportsmed,* June 41 (2), p. 67–74, 1993 (German)] and colleagues in 1993, subjects with different body types had interesting differences with respect to their hormone concentrations. For example, subjects with mesomorphic body types tended to have higher concentrations of testosterone and growth hormone, subjects with endomorphic body types tended to have higher concentrations of insulin, and subjects with ectomorphic body types tended to have higher concentrations of the hormone T3.

Keeping this discussion relevant to ectomorphs, the suggestion that T3, a potent thyroid hormone, is related to ectomorphy is interesting considering that clinical excesses of thyroid hormone can lead to the following:

» Increased metabolic rate and body temperature

» Increased appetite (but in some cases, the opposite can be true)

» Weight loss (with losses in lean tissue)

» Difficulty gaining muscle mass

» Difficulty sleeping

» Nervousness (also potential hand tremors)

» Inability to sit still

» Increased bowel movements and urination

» Decreased menstrual regularity (in women)

If it's true that some of the hypertrophy-challenged among you do have a bit more T3 floating around than your mesomorphic and/or endomorphic counterparts, you now have an explanation for your weight-gain woes. After all, unaccounted-for increases in resting metabolic rate, nervousness, fidgeting, and an inability to sit still can all increase daily energy expenditure (remember the RMR + NEAT calculation we did earlier), thus raising your energy requirements beyond even those we recommended earlier.

To compensate for the potential weight-gain resistance some of you may face, it should be clear that many of you are going to have to find ways to expend less total energy each day. That's right, you might actually have to, unlike most of your societal counterparts, become *more* sedentary. And, as we said earlier, you'll also need to find ways to ingest more total energy each day. That's right, the *more food* thing again. Now remember, while eating more and exercising less is what makes most of North America obese, in classic hypertrophy-challenged individuals, ectomorphs or otherwise, this prescription can actually improve health by increasing lean body mass, normalizing hormonal concentrations, and improving reproductive fitness.

But even the increasing-energy-intake part of the prescription presents a challenge to weight gain. If you're anything like the weight-gain-resistant subjects in the Levine study, even thousand-calorie increases in energy intake above maintenance may not be enough. Puzzling? Well, it shouldn't be after we discuss two more studies.

In a study published by Elliot Danforth Jr. and colleagues in *Journal of Clinical Investigation* (1979), overfeeding was shown to cause further increases in T3 concentrations, again increasing metabolism. Therefore if you have a bunch of extra T3 kicking around, and then you begin to overfeed, you might get a further boost in T3 concentrations. Considering the fact that Takashi Matsumoto and colleagues in *Obesity Research* (2001) demonstrated big increases in sympathetic nervous system activation after meals in lean subjects, if you're hypertrophy-challenged, already have high T3 concentrations, get a further T3 boost after eating, and get an increased sympathetic response to eating, you've got all the makings for a body stubborn to weight gain. Your fat friends now officially hate you!

But listen up, as we've been saying all along, just because you may be one of the few who has a more difficult time putting on weight, that doesn't mean that it's going to be impossible for you. To the contrary, follow our little tricks listed below, and what once seemed like a challenge will be nothing more than a puny obstacle in your rearview mirror.

INDIVIDUALIZING YOUR ENERGY INTAKE

After this last discussion, it's probably likely that most of you will just assume that you're the weight-gain-resistant type. However, don't jump to conclusions before you have empirical evidence. As we've discussed throughout the book, increasing muscle mass and muscle strength is an *outcome-based* pursuit. So start by following the training program recommended in the first section of the book and by using the calorie recommendations and menu plans listed in the second part of this book. For most of you, these will be enough to pack on muscle faster than David Banner after he gets angry (and you won't like him when he's angry). But just in case you turn out to be one of these hypertrophy-challenged guys who really can eat all day without gaining weight, *or* you turn out to be a little more weight-gain prone than you had imagined, we decided to provide a decision-making strategy that we use with our own one-on-one clients. By adopting this system, you can easily and systematically alter your energy intake to match your individual physiology.

The Decision-Making Matrix

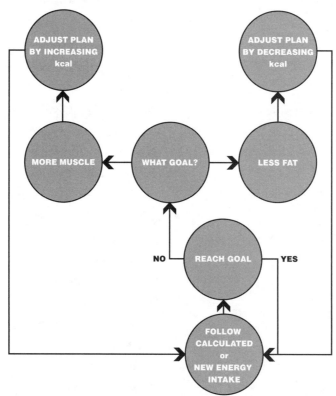

Here's how to use this decision-making strategy. After 2 weeks of following your nutritional plan (outlined in this book), it's time to assess your progress objectively (i.e., body weight and body-fat measurements). At this point, ask yourself whether you've accomplished your body composition goals (the "Reach Goal?" section of the chart above). If the answer is "Yes," simply keep repeating the plan as it now stands (until, of course, the answer becomes "No"). If, and/or when, the answer is/or becomes "No," then it's time for a change.

If your goal is to increase muscle mass (as we imagine it is for most of you), you need to adjust the original plan by eating more food. But don't just throw foods in randomly. Rather, you want to slowly begin the adjustment process by adding 250 kcal to your total daily energy intake.

If our example 200-pound guy from earlier were eating 3,800 kcal and not seeing the weight gain he wanted, he would simply increase his energy intake to 4,050 kcal (3,800 kcal + 250 kcal). If you're wondering what type of food to add in, sit tight; we'll cover that in the next chapter.

After making this 250-kcal adjustment, it's time to follow this adjustment for another 2 weeks. At the end of the 2 weeks, it's time for another reassessment of your goals. After recording body weight and measuring body fat, again ask yourself the question, "Reach Goals?" If the answer is "Yes," then keep repeating the plan as it now stands until the answer becomes "No." If the answer is "No," simply revisit the original plan, alter it by adding another 250 kcal to the total energy intake, and reassess after another 2 weeks.

By continuing on in this fashion, you'll easily be able to either gain weight or lose weight based on your goals. Seems pretty simple, right? Well, *the principle is simple.* The hard part comes in being patient enough to consistently follow the plan. If you can patiently and systematically follow this process (i.e., make an adjustment, wait 2 weeks, reassess, adjust again),

you'll find your patience is rewarded by steadily increasing muscle gains or fat loss. And herein lies the beauty of the system: You can follow it right up until the time you reach your goal. Then, by using the same readjustment process, you can follow it in your quest for a new goal, whether that's gaining another 10 pounds of body mass or whether it's losing body fat.

As the title of this chapter dictates, your weapon is a fork. In this day and age, with experts constantly promoting novel macronutrient ratios and fancy supplements, it's easy to lose sight of the most important determinant of body mass and body composition change—total energy intake. And total energy intake is directly proportional to the amount of times you raise your fork to your mouth.

While creatine supplementation helps some people gain a few pounds, it won't make you bigger unless you've already provided enough energy through your diet. And while the 40-30-30 ratios of the Zone Diet can produce great results in terms of fat loss or muscle gain, in the absence of an appropriate energy deficit or surplus, the Zone Diet will fall flat on its face. So take a lesson from the fact that we've devoted this entire chapter to calculating your energy needs and fine-tuning them. Your total energy intake is going to be the most important thing to get right about your nutrition. Don't make the same mistakes other scrawny guys make; don't undereat. Give those bricklayers their bricks.

In the next chapter, a chapter devoted to understanding the concept of nutrient timing and using it to give you the muscle-building edge that your friends don't have, we'll discuss how to spread your calorie intake out most effectively. After all, at this point, we've discussed only how many calories you need to eat per day. And certainly you'll get different results if you eat all of those in one sitting (can you say Sumo?) versus spreading them out over the course of the day. So check out Chapter 14 for the next step in planning your nutritional intake.

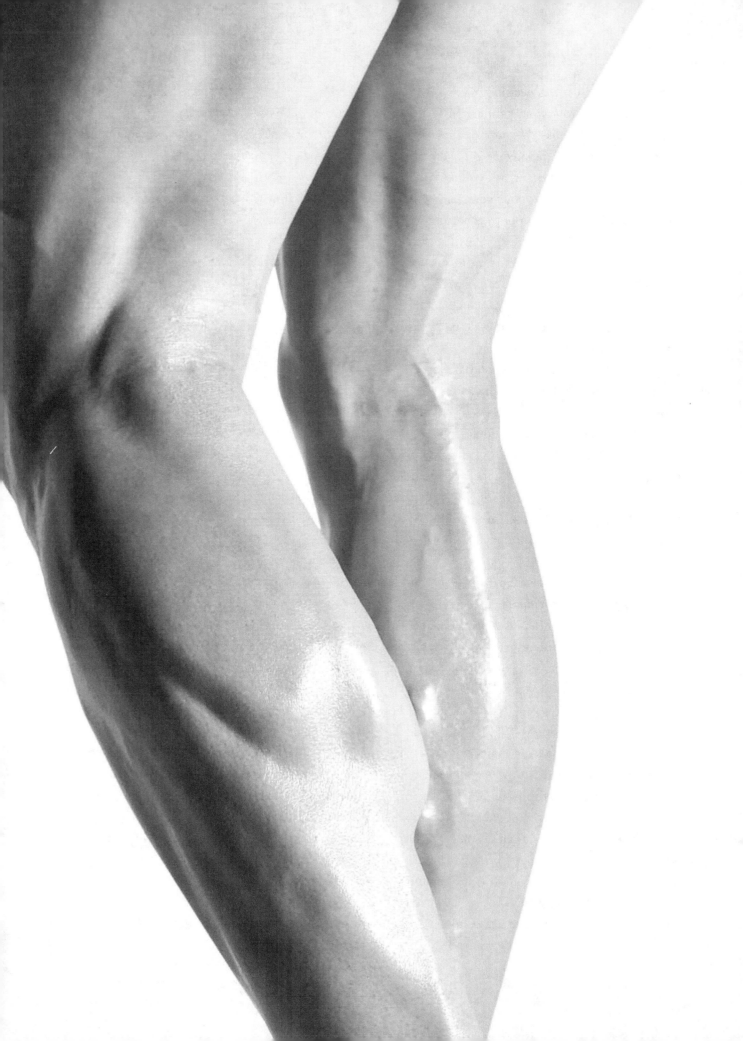

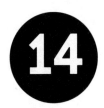

IT'S ALL ABOUT THE TIMING

》》 When planning your nutritional program, there are three critical questions you need to ask:

1. How much should I eat?

2. When should I eat all this food?

3. What should I eat at those times?

Answer these three questions effectively, and your days as a body double for Pee-Wee Herman are over. In Chapter 13, we covered how much you should be eating, providing you with activity-based calculations and making specific recommendations for adjusting these in an outcome-based manner, the outcome being your rate of physical change. However, we determined only *how much* you need to eat. In this chapter, we'll discuss nutrient timing including *when* you should eat all this food and *what* you should eat *at these specific times.*

When talking shop with conventional nutritionists, discussions about eating for body composition management, muscle building, and athletic performance usually center on *how much* to eat. However, despite the importance of eating more energy than you expend in gaining weight, this conventional *thermodynamic* approach to weight change tells just a portion of the story. After all, very few people would benefit from focusing exclusively on weight gain or weight loss. Rather, the focus should be on the *composition* of the gain or loss.

A focus on only weight gain or loss exclusively can lead to an overall disappointment in your nutrition plan. Although this might be a bit of an oversimplification of a very complex topic, in some ways the thermodynamic approach of measuring calories in versus calories out may simply maintain the body shape status quo (if there is such a thing). For example, if you're blessed with the right genetics, the calorie in versus calorie out thermodynamic approach to weight gain (or loss) will probably be all you need to look good *sans* clothes at any body size (bigger or smaller). In essence, you'll gain muscle at a faster rate than fat when trying to "bulk up," or you'll lose fat at a faster rate than muscle when trying to "lean out."

But what if you're not among the genetic elite? Well, simply eating more than you expend or eating less than you expend can just lead to equal gains or losses in fat and muscle, making you just a bigger or smaller version of your former self. So if you fall into this latter category and are also unhappy with that shape, you'll probably be unhappy if you try to change your energy balance alone.

And that's just body composition change. The traditional thermodynamic approach really doesn't address health in any significant way, either. The thermodynamic approach states that "a calorie is a calorie," and if you simply eat less than you expend (whatever you're eating), you'll lose weight. And if you eat more than you expend (whatever you're eating), you'll gain weight. Unfortunately, this approach doesn't differentiate between cottage cheese and Cheez Whiz, fat-free milk and Milk Duds, apples and apple pie.

To address some of the limitations of the thermodynamic or "calorie balance" approach presented above, scientists have begun to study the effects of different foods on body composition. Now we're not talking about the grapefruit diet here! Instead, we're talking about eating similar amounts of carbohydrate, just switching from a high-sugar diet to a diet low in sugar yet full of fruits and vegetables as well as low-glycemic-index grains. Other manipulations include replacing some saturated fat with monounsaturated fats such as olive oil or polyunsaturated fats such as fish oil. Through this research, scientists have found that once energy balance is accounted for, and you're eating more than you're expending when trying to gain weight, or eating less than you're expending

when trying to lose weight, the carbohydrates, proteins, and fats you choose can either help or hinder your composition changes. In essence, some carbohydrates are better than others because they better control the entry of sugar into your blood, moderating your insulin levels and leading to less fat gain. Some proteins are better than others because different proteins have different rates of entry into the bloodstream, and these properties, if utilized at the right times of the day, can improve your quest for new brawn. And some fats are better than others because certain fats can actually speed up your metabolism, increase testosterone production, and increase the amount of fat you burn. Therefore, by choosing your food wisely and eating the right foods at the right times, even if you're eating the same number of calories each day, you can effectively alter the composition of your weight gain and weight loss, and you'll reap the health benefits of a better diet composition.

As you can see, the science of *what* to eat has added to the *how much* to eat picture and advanced our understanding of body composition manipulation and achieving optimal health. In recognizing the laws of thermodynamics and eating accordingly, we can set the stage for weight loss or weight gain. And by choosing our foods wisely, we wield the power to take control of what types of gains and losses we'll see. In some respects, the science of *what* to eat has given us the power to transcend some of our genetic "inclinations" (i.e., overall body shape and genetic health risks).

We've discussed the *how much* to eat and *what* to eat perspectives. Yet there's one newly emerging area of research that can further assist in taking control of your body composition, including your weight gain and weight loss efforts. The science of *when* to eat is called "nutrient timing" and is becoming an important part of effective nutritional planning.

So what's so special about *when* you eat? Well, there are two main principles driving the importance of nutrient timing.

1. Once you determine *how much* to eat, you'll need to split those meals up so that you're eating frequently, and you're eating for the activities you've just completed as well as the activities you're about to undertake. In doing this, you can dramatically improve your body composition without even changing your dietary composition or daily energy balance.

2. If you build upon the first principle by actually increasing your overall energy intake and choosing the right foods at the right times of the day, your success will be unparalleled.

Research by Dan Benardot, Ph.D., R.D., at Georgia State University, has suggested that frequent eating as well as eating for the specific activities you'll be participating in or already have participated in offers the following benefits:

❱❱ Improved glucose tolerance

❱❱ Decreased insulin response to meals

❱❱ Decreased blood cortisol concentrations

❱❱ Decreased serum lipids

❱❱ Decreased adipose tissue (the fancy word for fat)

❱❱ Maintenance of metabolic rate

In other words, the first principle of nutrient timing offers a number of health and body composition benefits. So, once you know *how much* to eat, you can begin designing your nutritional program by arranging frequent feedings with the largest meals coming during the most active parts

of your day such as before/during/and after your workout and/or during your workday if you've got an active job.

This type of focus on eating when active provides another benefit: It prevents binge eating behaviors. Binge eating usually comes after maintaining a low blood sugar for an extended period of time. Your brain gets so fed up with your lack of eating (or eating too much sugar) and forces you to binge. And when do most binges occur? At night, right? So by keeping the body well fed and the brain happy during the active parts of your day, you'll be much less likely to binge on crappy food choices at night.

With respect to the second principle of nutrient timing, it's important to realize that certain foods are good during certain times of the day, yet not so good during others. Sure, if your diet's pretty poor, and like many North Americans, you're eating too much sugar, too little fiber, and too much saturated fat relative to the other fats in your diet, a simple shift in what you eat will go a long way toward helping you manage your body composition and your health. But if you're really interested in packing on the muscle mass, it's important to understand that although sugar shouldn't make up the bulk of your dietary intake, there is a time and a place for it.

For example, simple carbohydrates like sugar are great during the postworkout recovery period but not so great outside this critical recovery period (see Chapter 13). Likewise, high-fiber foods are great during most meals of the day but are suboptimal during the immediate postexercise period. When speaking of protein, fast-digesting protein such as whey is great during the immediate postworkout period, but whey is not so great during the rest of the day. It's important to understand that, often, a natural food's value is based on when you eat it, not just its composition alone. Sure, there are *lots* of artificial foods that are completely bad for you (if a food's ingredients list contains the words hydrogenated or partially hydrogenated, or contains a bunch of big words you can't pronounce, it's likely the food contains a lot of artificial ingredients and should stay on the grocery store shelves), but a natural food's value can be based on when you eat it. Although this idea may be new to you, in the next few sections, we'll discuss why some foods are better than others at specific times of the day. By the end of this chapter, you should have a pretty firm grasp of which foods fit in where.

To understand why nutrient timing is so important to the athlete, it's important to understand these points:

1. Much of the current science is pointing to the fact that if you train regularly, during specific times of the day, the body is primed for fat gain or fat loss just as it's primed for muscle gain or muscle loss during other times of the day. Add in the wrong foods at the wrong times, and you're sabotaging your efforts in the gym. Add the right foods, and your efforts are given a giant boost.

2. Although some foods are not optimal during certain times of the day (i.e., sugar), some of these same foods can actually be very beneficial during other times of the day (such as the post-workout period).

In order to easily teach you the basics of which foods should be incorporated and when without writing an entire dissertation, we're going to break your training day down into four phases and teach you what you should be eating during each phase. The four phases are as follows:

Phase I: The Energy Phase

Phase II: The Anabolic Phase

Phase III: The Growth Phase

Phase IV: The Recovery Phase

Phase I is called the Energy Phase because this phase occurs during the workout when energy demands are highest. You see, the metabolic rate during intense weight training can be six to eight times higher than the metabolic rate at rest (there are those METs again). The breakdown products from carbohydrates, proteins, and fats provide the energy needed to sustain this increase in metabolic rate. These carbohydrates, proteins, and fats can come from either ingested food (food eaten immediately prior to exercise or during exercise) or from body stores of carbohydrate (muscle and liver glycogen), protein (muscle mass or the free amino acid pool), or fat (adipose tissue or intramuscular triglycerides). If you end up burning body stores, no surprise, you get smaller. Since that's the opposite of what we're trying to do, it's important to ingest the appropriate nutrients during training. If done properly, you'll definitely get bigger as long as your nutrition is adequate during the remainder of the day.

Based on new scientific research, targeted nutritional intake during Phase I can actually promote a series of positive benefits independent of the energy provision alone. Good nutrition during the Energy Phase can provide these benefits:

❱❱ Increase bloodflow to the working muscles

❱❱ Increase nutrient delivery to the working muscles

❱❱ Reduce muscle glycogen depletion

❱❱ Reduce the amount of muscle protein breakdown

❱❱ Decrease blood concentrations of the catabolic hormone cortisol (and this is good because cortisol can break down muscles)

❱❱ Improve immune function

» Shift the anabolic (muscle building)/catabolic (muscle breakdown) balance during exercise toward muscle building rather than breakdown (since breakdown/catabolism is usually predominant during most training sessions).

During the Energy Phase, we recommend drinking a liquid protein/carbohydrate supplement just prior to your workout (about 10 to 15 minutes before). In addition, you should be sipping another one during the workout. Since these supplements are in liquid form, if sipped throughout the workout, dehydration, a potent performance killer in both strength and endurance athletes, can be prevented as well. But just any old liquid protein/carbohydrate drinks won't do. Since the body needs those nutrients quickly, you've gotta pick rapidly digesting proteins and carbohydrates. Even a standard meal replacement powder drink can take up to an hour or more to be fully digested. Therefore, a drink containing simple sugar (sugar is quickly digested) and fast-digesting protein like whey protein is optimal.

The next nutrient timing phase we'd like to address is the Anabolic Phase. The Anabolic Phase occurs immediately after the workout and lasts about an hour or two. This phase is titled "anabolic" because it's during this time that the muscle cells are primed for muscle building (anabolism means "building," and in the case of muscle physiology, references to anabolic states or anabolism mean muscle building). Interestingly, though, although the cells are primed for muscle building after the workout (during the Anabolic Phase), in the absence of a good nutritional strategy, this phase can remain very catabolic (catabolism means "breakdown, and in the case of muscle physiology, references to catabolic states or catabolism mean muscle breakdown). So this phase becomes anabolic only when you make the right nutritional choices.

As mentioned, without adequate nutrition, the period immediately after strength and endurance training is marked by a net muscle catabolism; in other words, muscles continue to break down after exercise. Now, if you're asking yourself how this can be, you're asking the right question. After all, training (especially weight training) makes you bigger, not smaller. And even if you're an endurance athlete, your muscles don't exactly break down either. So how can exercise be so catabolic?

Well, for starters, while the few hours after exercise induce a net catabolic state (although protein synthesis does increase after exercise, so does breakdown), it's later in the recovery cycle that the body begins to shift toward anabolism. So we typically break down for some time after the workout and then start to build back up later (whether that "buildup" is in muscle size or in muscle quality). However, with this said, the use of liquid protein/carbohydrate supplements after training can actually help you improve your recovery and lead to a net increase in muscle size or quality during and immediately after exercise. So, with the right nutritional intake during the Anabolic Phase, you don't have to wait until the next day to start growing. You'll start growing right away.

To get the most out of the Anabolic Phase, you need to drink another liquid protein/carbohydrate supplement immediately after your workout (in addition to the one you'll be drinking prior to working out, and the one you'll be sipping during your workout). By doing so, you'll essentially be duplicating the benefits described earlier during Phase I, doubling or even tripling the effectiveness of your drink and further enhancing the anabolic effects of nutrition on muscle building and muscle glycogen recovery.

At this point, it's important to recognize that Phases I and II are marked by a dramatically increased anabolic potential. During and immediately after the workout, dietary amino acids and dietary carbohydrates (especially the rapidly digested kind) are most efficient in terms of their effects on muscle growth. For a grossly oversimplified description, picture it this way. If you eat 100 amino acids and 200 glucose units before, during, and after your workout, all 100 amino acids and 200 glucose units reach the muscle for energy provision, rebuilding, and recovery. However, if you eat those same 100 amino acids and 200 glucose units during the remainder of the day, only 50 amino acids and 100 glucose units will be used for muscle building, while the other 50 amino acids and 100 glucose units will be used for other purposes (including fat gain). So as you can see, after the workout, the body is much more efficient with those proteins and carbs you're feeding yourself. Of course, all the while you're keeping in mind the first premise of nutrient timing discussed earlier; you're eating for the activities you've just done as well as the activities you're about to do.

As a result of this increased exercise and postexercise efficiency, it should be clear that after your workout, you can load up on specific carbohydrates and proteins that might normally be counterproductive. After all, sugar is a no-no outside the workout and postworkout periods but is one of the best types of food to ingest during the workout and postworkout periods. Again, it's not about food being necessarily good or bad. A food is only as good or bad as the time you eat it. Using the proper application of nutrient timing, the right kinds of foods should be eaten when they'll best improve the body. And the most important time to consider doing so is during this exercise and postexercise "anabolic window" occurring during Phases I and II.

But since the "anabolic window" is "open" only for a short period of time, it's important to quickly feed the drinks listed above and then begin to prepare for the next phase, Phase III. Phase III, the Growth Phase, begins about 2 to 3 hours after your

workout and is characterized by a return to normal metabolism.

After protein and carbohydrate have been provided during the Energy and Anabolic Phases and the net protein balance of the body shifted toward the positive, muscle glycogen restored, catabolism blunted, and anabolism increased, it's time to consider how to keep the growth process moving forward. After all, the muscle damage from your workout has been done, and your metabolism is going to be racing until the next day. Of course, as you should now realize, if the metabolism is up, it's time to eat more.

However, even though the body is under construction, it's moving quickly back toward normal functioning as that anabolic window closes. With this slow return to "normalcy," it's important to ditch the sugary, high-glycemic carbohydrates and rapidly digested proteins recommended above (and in Chapter 13). While these foods were the anabolic superstars of the Energy and Anabolic Phases, you'll have to thank them and send them on their merry way during Phase III: the Growth Phase and Phase IV: the Recovery Phase. These drinks provide a big, muscle-building insulin surge (insulin is a very anabolic hormone), so they're beneficial during and after exercise. But elevate the insulin all day, and your reward will be a chubby midsection.

Starting about 3 hours after your workout, there is a distinct challenge. While the body's efficiency at restoring muscle glycogen and taking up amino acids for growth was heightened just after the workout, it's now back to normal, and the anabolic window is closed. This would be fine if the muscle had completely recovered during this time. However, your muscles may still be partially depleted (especially the ones you just trained) and will certainly be damaged for another couple of days. So at this point, it's critical to eat enough total food to compensate for the increased metabolism accompanying the Growth Phase, enough carbohydrate to resynthesize muscle glycogen, and enough protein to repair the muscle damage you caused during training. As you might expect, during the Growth Phase, it's important to continue to feed some carbohydrate and protein. But at this time, the key is to begin to reduce the total amount of carbohydrates ingested per meal while increasing the amount of protein ingested per meal. While ingesting 2 grams of carbohydrate to every 1 gram of protein was optimal for the Energy and Anabolic Phases, you should strive for a 1:1 ratio now. You could even throw in a little dietary fat with these meals as long as the meals remain predominantly P + C (protein plus carbohydrate).

Also, during the Growth Phase, you're going to start chewing real food rather than slurping down drinks. Real food is more slowly digested and absorbed, and while this isn't optimal for the workout and postworkout periods, this is optimal for the Growth Phase. Quick-digesting nutrition at this time would increase insulin concentrations and cause unmanageable fluctuations in blood sugar and amino acids, leading to energy swings and even excess fat gain. So it's important to choose slower-digesting proteins (meats, cottage cheese, yogurt, etc.) and low-glycemic carbohydrates (fruits, vegetables, beans, oats, wild rice, ancient grains such as quinoa, etc.) during the Growth Phase.

Since the Growth Phase lasts about 3 to 4 hours, you should be able to fit about two protein/carbohydrate meals (with a 1:1 ratio of slower digesting protein and low-glycemic-index carbohydrate) here.

So let's tally up our meal recommendations so far. For those of you keeping score, the Energy, Anabolic, and Growth Phases cover about 7 or 8 hours of your training day. During these 7 to 8 hours, you'll be ingesting about five total meals: two liquid supplements during the Energy Phase, and one liquid supplement during the Anabolic Phase (each supplement containing approximately a 2:1 ratio of protein to carbohydrate), and two

during the Growth Phase (each meal containing approximately a 1:1 ratio of protein to carbohydrate). The first three meals contain protein and carbohydrate with no fat while the last two meals may contain small amounts of dietary fat, making all five meals P + C meals.

As noted in the previous chapter, we separate meals into what we call P + C, or protein plus carbohydrate, meals and P + F, or protein plus fat, meals. A P + C meal contains predominantly protein and carbohydrate with little fat. A P + F meal contains predominantly protein and fat with little carbohydrate.

While the idea of eating this way may seem odd to some readers, removing much of the fat from P + C meals and much of the carbohydrate from P + F meals is a great way to add muscle mass without adding excess body fat (as long as the P + C and P + F meals are eaten at the right times).

Once the Energy, Anabolic, and Growth Phases are covered, assuming you sleep about 8 hours per day, that leaves 8 to 9 hours and three meals to complete your dietary intake. It's these 8 to 9 hours and three meals that we consider Phase IV, or the Recovery Phase.

Since the Recovery Phase is marked by normal physiology, and you should have replenished much of your muscle glycogen during the previous three phases, the Recovery Phase should be full of protein and the healthy fats that weren't ingested during the previous three phases. As indicated earlier, P + C meals are warranted during certain times of the day. However, P + F meals, or protein plus fat meals, are also necessary during other parts of the day, namely during the Recovery Phase. To optimize your recovery phase meals, these feedings should contain quality proteins as well as an equal blend of saturated fats, monounsaturated fats, and polyunsaturated fats. But don't avoid carbohydrates altogether. Just choose vegetables and a small amount of fruit during these meals.

NUTRIENT TIMING BY PHASE

PHASE	TIMING	MEAL TYPE	RATIO
Phase I: The Energy Phase	10 minutes before training	Liquid P + C	2:1 (carbohydrate to protein, no fat)
	Sip during training	Liquid P + C	2:1 (carbohydrate to protein, no fat)
Phase II: The Anabolic Phase	Immediately after training	Liquid P + C	2:1 (carbohydrate to protein, no fat)
Phase III: The Growth Phase	1 hour after training	P + C	1:1 (carbohydrate to protein, little fat)
	3 hours after training	P + C	1:1 (carbohydrate to protein, little fat)
Phase IV: The Recovery Phase	Three or four meals during the remainder of the day	All P + F	From 1:1 to 2:1 (protein to fat, little carb)

In checking out the table above, some basic organizational questions may arise, like what if someone trains in the evening? Well, the principles of nutrient timing are similar no matter what. Below, we've provided a handy table detailing how you might apply this system if you work out during the morning, afternoon, or evening. Remember, though, these can be tweaked subtly to accommodate your schedule.

SCHEDULING YOUR MEALS AROUND WORKOUTS

MORNING WORKOUT (6:00–7:30 AM)	AFTERNOON WORKOUT (12:00–1:30 PM)	EVENING WORKOUT (6:00–7:30 PM)
5:45 AM Liquid P + C	6:00–6:30 AM P + F	6:00–6:30 AM P + C
6:00–7:30 AM Liquid P + C	9:00–9:30 AM P + F	9:00–9:30 AM P + F
7:30 AM Liquid P + C	11:45 AM Liquid P + C	12:00–12:30 PM P + F
9:30–10:00 AM P + C	12:00–1:30 PM Liquid P + C	3:00–3:30 PM P + F
12:30–1:00 PM P + C	1:30 PM Liquid P + C	5:45 PM Liquid P + C
4:00–4:30 PM P + F	3:30–4:00 PM P + C	6:00–7:30 PM Liquid P + C
6:30–7:00 PM P + F	6:00–6:30 PM P + C	7:30 PM Liquid P + C
9:30–10:00 PM P + F	9:00–9:30 PM P + F	9:30–10:00 PM P + C

Again, this nutrient timing idea might be a bit strange sounding at first. But one interesting way of looking at your food consumption during a "nutrient timing day" is such that you're eating like Atkins Diet proponents might recommend during three of your meals (the Recovery Phase), like Zone Diet proponents might recommend during two of your meals (the Growth Phase), and like the American Dietetics Association might recommend during three more of your meals (the Energy and Anabolic Phases). Of course, this system wasn't designed solely to reconcile the three big dietary movements but rather to use what we currently know about exercise metabolism to meet your daily energy needs in order to optimize growth, adaptation, performance, and body composition.

Obviously, our nutrient timing discussion has focused on eating around your workouts. So the guidelines above are for application on training days. But what about off days? Well, during your off days, you should be eating the same way as during training days, only you'll be eliminating the three liquid drinks ingested during the Anabolic and Growth Phases. In doing so, you'll easily be able to eliminate a few hundred calories (remember, your total energy expenditure is smaller on non-training days) without even missing them.

At this point, you should be able to come up with basic answers to the big three questions:

1. *How much* should I eat?

2. *When* should I eat all this food?

3. *What* should I eat *at those times*?

By eating frequently, eating for upcoming activities or activities already performed, and introducing certain foods when they are most needed by the body, your days of being hypertrophy-challenged are numbered.

Now, before moving on to Chapter 15, a chapter discussing workout nutrition, we want to address an objection that has undoubtedly surfaced. We know that many of you are reading this and thinking that these last two chapters have been pretty detail oriented and in all this detail lay some serious challenges to your current lifestyle. After all, many of you are eating only three meals per day right now (plus a protein bar or shake or two if you're lucky). And here we come, suggesting five full-food meals and three shakes on training days. That seems like an awful lot of meals to get down every day, doesn't it?

But as discussed earlier, it's our job to be honest and up front about what it's going to take to reach your brawny goals. If you're someone who thinks this meal plan is unrealistic for your unique scenario, we're not going to tell you to just tough it out. However, we are going to tell you that it can be done. We are going to tell you that this plan is possible for you even if you're the "average guy" who spends 8 to 10 hours a day running around at the office. If you're thinking that only people who have nothing to do but eat and exercise all day long can follow this . . . Wait a second, do you hear that? That's right, our BS detectors just went off.

Listen, it's time for some tough love. For starters, we know the objections that are bound to come up because we've been guilty of thinking them. When we were scrawny ourselves, we uttered the same excuses. But nowadays, you won't hear them from us despite the fact that we're two of the busiest guys around. You see, nearly everyone is busy. Some are "too busy" to do those home renovation projects they've been meaning to get to, some are "too busy" to contact an old friend, some are "too busy" to work on the proposal that might just guarantee their financial security, and some are "too busy" to finally start taking control of their health and body composition. Yet somehow others in their very same position find a way to get it done.

So what's the difference between these two types? Those who succeed find solutions to their time-management challenges while those who don't succeed find excuses. So next time you begin to waste time finding "too busy" excuses, realize that your time would be better spent finding ways to fit positive habits, such as the principles of nutrient timing, into your schedule. In Chapter 15, we'll present some strategies for helping you do so.

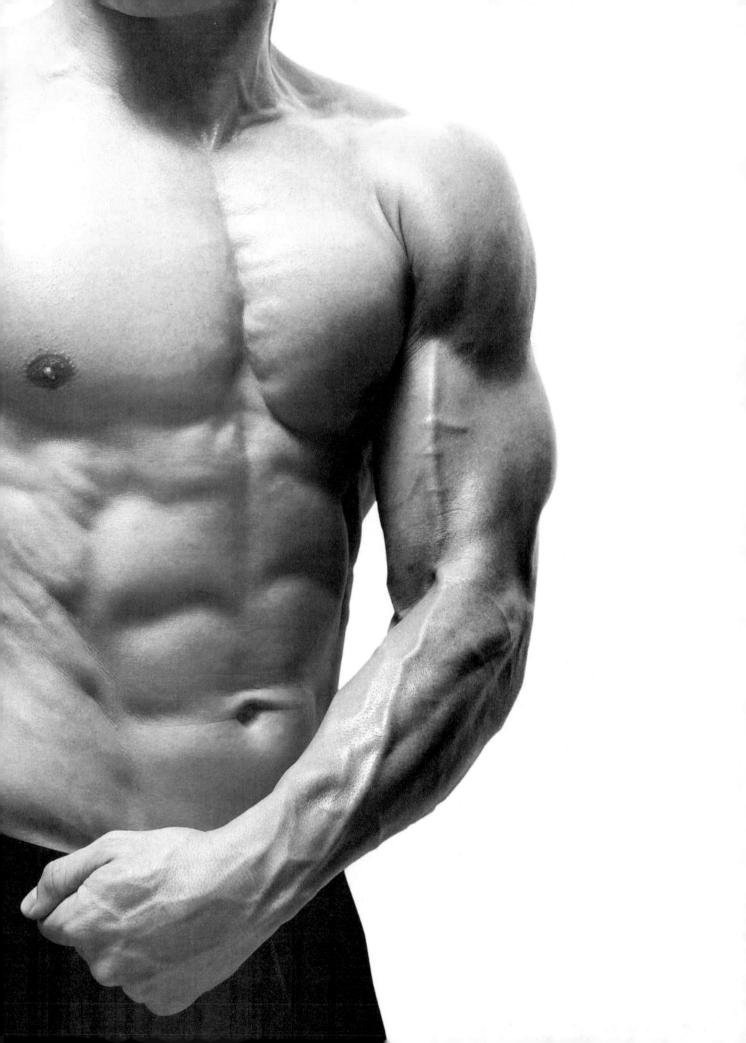

WORKOUT NUTRITION

» A big part of the nutrient timing concept addressed in the previous chapter is the idea that if you want to grow, you've got to be drinking specific nutrients during Phases I and II of nutrient timing, the Energy and Anabolic Phases. And no, beer does not constitute "specific nutrients."

In Chapter 13, we addressed the critical importance of eating an abundance of energy. We maintained that total energy intake is the most important determinant of your progress. But once your energy needs are covered, and you're getting all the vitamins and minerals necessary for optimal function, the next step in becoming a master of gaining mass is to optimize your preworkout, workout, and postworkout nutrition. Since workout nutrition is so critical a topic, even though we've briefly addressed it in the previous chapter, we've decided to use this chapter to expand upon this idea so that you can get an idea of why.

As discussed earlier, weight training causes an almost immediate six- to eightfold increase in metabolic activity. It's the dramatic increase in muscle energy utilization that creates the fundamental driving force for many of the physiological changes that occur during and after weight-training exercise. In the table on page 196, we've listed the predominant changes that occur during weight training.

As you can see in the table, there are both favorable changes and unfavorable changes that occur with exercise. Most unfortunately, for a short period of time during and after training, the balance is shifted toward the unfavorable side. That's right, the catabolic (potentially muscle-shrinking) processes initiated during training outweigh the anabolic (potential muscle-building) processes.

Before current research taught us otherwise, people assumed that they simply had to take the good with the bad and ride out the catabolic wave until anabolism started up again, hours into the recovery period. Fortunately now, we know otherwise. Scientists have found that we can use specific nutritional protocols to target the catabolic properties of exercise and minimize their damage. Later in this chapter, we'll discuss these nutritional protocols. However, prior to doing so, we want you to become familiar with exactly what's happening during the workout and postworkout periods.

As specified in the chart above, without targeted nutritional intervention, catabolism can dominate during the Energy Phase. In addition, as a result of the events that are initiated during the workout, the Anabolic Phase can be marked by the following:

1. Low/depleted muscle glycogen stores

2. Elevated protein breakdown rates

3. Negative shifts in muscle protein balance

As a consequence of these phenomena, a failure to rapidly bring the body back into recovery mode presents several practical problems:

1. Prolonged muscle soreness and fatigue

2. Poor subsequent performances in the gym

3. Symptoms of and/or full-fledged staleness, leading to overtraining

4. Minimal gains of muscle mass despite a good training program

5. Losses of muscle mass

6. A secondary lowering of metabolic rate

As discussed in the previous chapter, these outcomes might seem a bit confusing since we're sure that you know a lot of people who've gotten bigger from training with weights, yet these same people haven't really done much to improve their nutritional intake. So to eliminate the confusion, it's important to understand the time course of recovery following weight training.

Back in 1995, Canadian researchers demonstrated that immediately after strength training, muscle protein balance is negative (indicating some degree of muscle loss during this time). This negative muscle protein balance is due to a big increase in protein breakdown in the face of a very small increase in protein synthesis after training. Furthermore, while we call this postworkout phase the Anabolic Phase, without adequate postexercise nutrition, this period could easily turn into a catabolic nightmare.

While the body is inclined to be catabolic for a few hours after training, fortunately, a few hours later, an interesting switch occurs. Hours after training, protein synthesis starts to climb, and breakdown starts to fall (although it's still elevated above what's seen at rest). And this shift continues until about 24 hours later, when the muscle protein balance becomes positive. Here, protein synthesis is finally greater than protein breakdown, and on come those muscle gains you knew were supposed to arrive. It's only the first few hours after the workout that are extremely catabolic. Twenty-four

ANABOLIC AND CATABOLIC CHANGES THAT OCCUR WITH EXERCISE

ANABOLIC EFFECTS OF EXERCISE

Increased skeletal muscle bloodflow (improves nutrient delivery)

Increased anabolic hormone release (GH, Testosterone, IGF-1)

Acute phase response (after catabolic phase, muscle is rebuilt with improvements)

CATABOLIC EFFECTS OF EXERCISE

Muscle glycogen depletion (reduction of muscle carbohydrates)

Decreased protein balance (net loss of protein when subtracting protein synthesis and protein breakdown)

Increased cortisol concentrations (cortisol is a catabolic hormone)

Decreased insulin concentrations (insulin is an anabolic hormone)

Acute phase response (causes breakdown of damaged and some undamaged muscle tissue)

Increased metabolic rate (more nutrient depletion)

Dehydration (caused during training in the heat)

hours later, the body has normalized itself and becomes anabolic. But remember, until you hit that 24-hour mark, the muscles you trained are headed in the wrong direction. So how do you get them back on track?

Well, for starters, you've gotta optimize your intake during the Energy Phase. Scientists at the University of Texas at Galveston have demonstrated that a protein/carbohydrate supplement ingested immediately prior to exercise (within 15 minutes of beginning) can actually increase skeletal muscle bloodflow beyond what occurs during training already. Now, since this drink will contain amino acids (the building blocks of protein) and glucose (the building blocks of glycogen), this increased bloodflow will be full of nutrients that assist in muscle performance during the workout and assist in recovery after the workout.

What's exciting about this is the fact that while the catabolic events discussed earlier are still taking place during training, the nutrients floating around in your blood can promote such a rapid recovery that very little muscle breakdown actually occurs during the workout. In fact, data from the lab in Texas have demonstrated that the net effect of drinking a liquid protein/carbohydrate supplement right before training is an anabolic one. So in their subjects, muscle was actually built during training. Until this study was conducted, most experts would have thought that this was impossible.

As you should now be seeing, a simple preworkout protein/carbohydrate supplement can help reverse the catabolic cascade. Now, while a single preworkout supplement will probably go a long way toward helping prevent excess muscle breakdown, our trainees often go a step or two further by also sipping a protein/carbohydrate supplement during their actual weight-training workout. In doing so, in addition to helping shift protein balance to a more positive state, research has shown that these supplements can reduce muscle glycogen depletion, decrease those catabolic cortisol concentrations, improve the overall immune response

to exercise, and provide more energy/calories at a time when they are needed most, your most active period of the day. Remember the rules of nutrient timing. Eat frequently, and eat for the activities you've just done as well as the activities you're about to do.

So by using our preworkout and during workout nutrition suggestions, you'll prevent that muscle-shrinking negative protein balance, you'll prevent muscle glycogen depletion, you'll fight off the nasty catabolic hormone cortisol, and you'll be less likely to get sick. Of course, since the aforementioned supplements will be in liquid form and will be ingested both before exercise and sipped during the exercise bout, dehydration, a potent performance killer in both strength and endurance athletes, can be staved off as well. Not too shabby for a simple drink containing some protein and carbohydrate.

So up until this point, we've taken you through both the preworkout and the workout periods or the Anabolic Phase. Next, it's time to discuss the postworkout period or the Energy Phase. The goals of the postworkout period are similar to those we're hoping to accomplish during the workout itself.

1. Rapidly replenish the low glycogen stores in our muscles. Glycogen replenishment (refilling muscle glycogen stores) is important for maintaining peak performance because glycogen provides a rapid and readily available energy source for exercise performance, for preventing energy-related losses in muscle mass, for increasing cellular hydration, and for preventing rising concentrations of blood cortisol.

2. Rapidly decrease the muscle protein breakdown that occurs with exercise and further enhance muscle protein synthesis. By rapidly increasing protein synthesis while simultaneously decreasing protein breakdown, postworkout nutrition can shift your body toward a positive muscle protein balance within 1 hour after the workout. Did you get that? With proper postworkout nutrition, your muscle protein status may return to normal in within 1 hour. Remember we said earlier that typically a trainee has to wait 24 hours for a positive muscle protein balance? Using recovery nutrition, you can recover nearly a day earlier than you otherwise would have!

With these considerations in mind, in order to drive the body toward muscle building during the postworkout period, it's time to ingest another liquid protein/carbohydrate supplement. That's right, we're recommending three liquid protein/carbohydrate supplements. You should be drinking one within 15 minutes of your workout, sipping one during your workout, and drinking one final drink within 15 minutes of finishing your workout.

Why so soon after the workout? Well, the research is very clear that if you wait to consume your postworkout nutrition, you lose. One study showed that if the postworkout beverage was consumed immediately after training, glycogen synthesis was three times higher than if the beverage was consumed just 2 hours later.

But will any old protein/carbohydrate supplement do? Well, any old liquid protein/carbohydrate supplement is certainly better than nothing. But specific nutrients can offer specific advantages in terms of glycogen resynthesis and protein balance. Here's why.

To begin with, there are two key factors to rapidly increasing postworkout glycogen synthesis:

1. Providing an adequate carbohydrate intake

2. Stimulating high blood concentrations of the anabolic hormone insulin, a hormone that shuttles carbohydrates into the muscle for glycogen storage

Although conventional sports nutrition advice suggests that athletes ingest large amounts of carbohydrate alone, recent evidence indicates that the addition of protein to a carbohydrate drink can actually increase insulin concentrations more than carbohydrate alone. There seems to be a synergistic insulin release with a drink containing protein and carbohydrate.

Our current recommendation, then, includes the ingestion of 0.8 g carbohydrate per kg of body mass and 0.4 g protein per kg of body mass. This means that a 70 kg (or 154-pound) guy should be ingesting 56 g of carbs and 28 g of protein for each of his three protein carbohydrate supplements.

With respect to the types of carbohydrate and protein to consume, it's clear that immediately after training, liquid nutrition is best tolerated. Since liquid nutrition is more rapidly digested and absorbed, nutrients are more rapidly delivered to the muscle. For the most rapid response, the best types of carbohydrate to ingest are simple glucose and glucose polymers such as maltodextrin. Both can be purchased cheaply on the Internet and are also available in most commercial recovery formulas.

You want to choose a protein that is absorbed as rapidly as the glucose and glucose polymers we suggested. If the protein and carbohydrates are absorbed at a similar rate, the synergistic insulin response that we're expecting is maximized. Unfortunately, a protein source that's digested as quickly as glucose is hard to find. Most intact proteins (yes, even powdered forms of relatively fast-digesting proteins such as whey concentrates or isolates) are slower than ideal. Whey concentrates or isolates can take 1 to 2 hours to reach maximum concentrations. Since we need a protein that can get absorbed within minutes, just like the glucose/glucose polymers, we need to choose something even faster. Whey hydrolysates (otherwise known as hydrolyzed whey protein) are perfect for this function. And whey hydrolysates are not only fast; they're non-allergenic. Even people with mild milk protein intolerances or lactose intolerance can handle hydrolyzed whey protein. You'll know if you've got an intolerance if you get gassy, bloated, or congested after drinking your regular protein supplement.

These ingredients also do a good job of suppressing protein breakdown. Several studies within the past few years have demonstrated that insulin is the main regulator of postworkout protein breakdown. Therefore the synergistic insulin release promoted by the protein/carbohydrate combination discussed above is a good start toward suppressing protein breakdown. However, to really crank up the insulin production during the postworkout period, it's important to add in a few grams of amino acids on top of the amino acids in the whey protein. Research in the 1960s showed that specific amino-acid combinations were more effective than others at increasing insulin release. We've found that the best combination of amino acids and protein to promote an insulin response is a combination of hydrolyzed whey protein, a few grams of the branched chain amino acids (BCAA) leucine, isoleucine, and valine, a few grams of glutamine, and a few grams of phenylalanine.

Once glycogen resynthesis is maximized and protein breakdown minimized, the final consideration is managing protein synthesis. Although this goal is a little more complex than managing protein breakdown, there are three key ingredients to increasing protein synthesis immediately after workouts:

1. A proper ratio of BCAAs

2. High blood concentrations of essential amino acids

3. High blood concentrations of insulin

Several studies have shown that either infused (delivered via an intravenous drip) or orally administered postworkout amino acids are able to rapidly increase protein synthesis as well as rapidly create a positive muscle protein balance after training. In addition, BCAAs seem to play a big role in the recovery and the increase of protein synthesis after a workout. And, of course, we already know how to increase insulin concentrations.

So in the end, the Energy and Anabolic Phases are the two most critical phases in the nutrient timing system. During the workout and just after, the body is primed for efficient nutrient uptake and recovery. By using what we know about muscle glycogen storage and recovery, muscle protein balance, and hormonal status, we can manipulate workout nutrition to produce some pretty amazing results. The following table presents a list of ingredients and the times that you should take them. Remember, for optimal results, use as directed below. Several commercial recovery drinks are available and contain this ideal composition. In addition, you can easily obtain the ingredients online and mix up your own home brew. Unfortunately, yours isn't likely to taste as good.

WORKOUT NUTRITION FOR MAXIMAL RESULTS

	PREWORKOUT (WITHIN 15 MINUTES OF EXERCISE)	DURING WORKOUT (SIP DURING)	POSTWORKOUT (IMMEDIATELY AFTER)
Carbohydrate	0.8 g/kg	0.8 g/kg	0.8 g/kg
Protein	0.4 g/kg	0.4 g/kg	0.4 g/kg
Fat	0 g	0 g	0 g
Amino Acids			
BCAA	~3–5 g	~3–5 g	~3–5 g
Glutamine	~3 g	~3 g	~3 g
Phenylalanine	~3–5 g	~3 g	~3 g

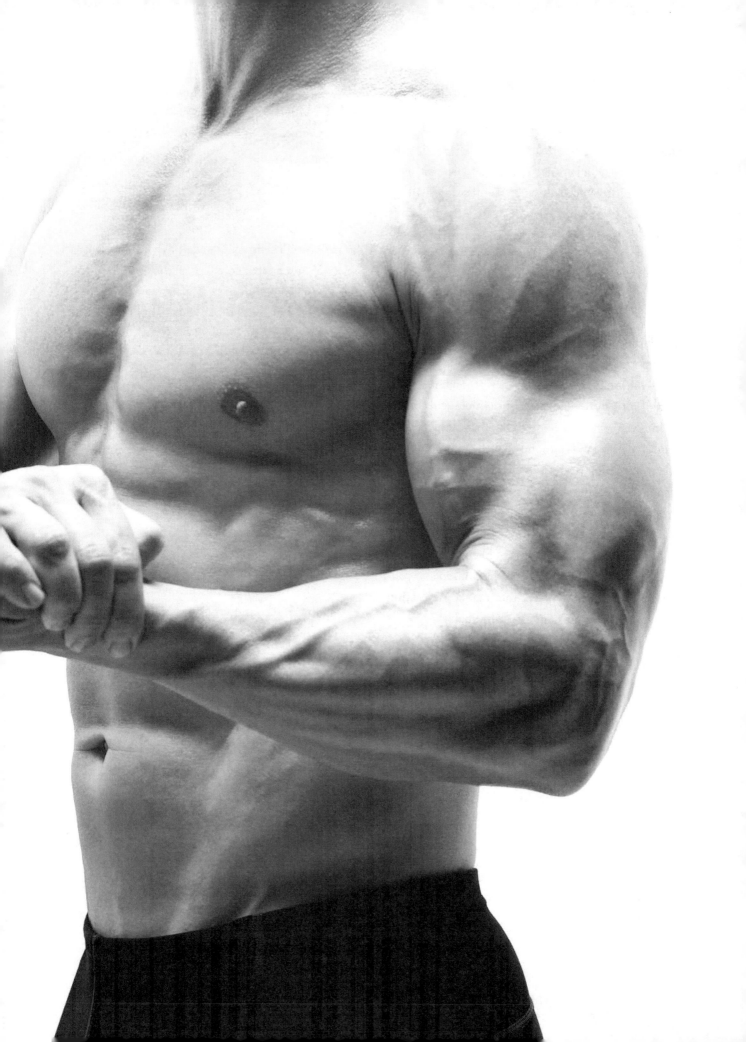

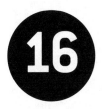

SUPPLEMENTS AND THE
HYPERTROPHY-CHALLENGED

》》If we were to guess, we might presume that this is the chapter many
of you have anxiously anticipated. That's right, not even we can totally resist the idea that there might be some supplemental pill, powder, or potion that
gives us an extra edge when we're consistently training hard and eating well. Sure, the
supplement naysayers will mock this as looking for the "magic pill." But those of us who
know better remain unmoved by their cynicism. Little do they know that there are a few
supplements that, when taken as an adjunct to an excellent program, do give us a small
but measurable boost in the gym while actually improving our health. Wanting this edge
isn't lazy or foolhardy. It's completely rational. To us, it's irrational to ignore potentially
beneficial compounds designed to make those hours we spend in the gym more effective, dismissing them all with but a snicker (and then going to eat a Snickers bar!).

Now, on the opposite side of the coin, there may be a few of you out there hoping
that there actually is a magic pill that can help you build muscle while allowing you to
only half-heartedly attempt the training and nutritional modifications suggested
throughout the book. For those of you who believe this, uh . . . Mike . . . please put
down the gun . . .

Uh, as we were saying, for those of you who actually believe this, we're going to expose this fraudulent idea right now. So listen up. There are no legal supplements that
can help you build muscle in the absence of a well-planned and consistently adhered-to
training and nutritional program. In other words, supplements work toward building
muscle only when they're taken in addition to a training program designed to ensure
maximal adaptation and a nutritional program designed to provide an abundance of
energy. Trying to add a bunch of supplements into a crappy program is the equivalent
of adding a nitrous system to a broken-down Pinto. No matter how much you spend on
modifications, the car isn't going anywhere.

Even with the "very powerful" supplements (i.e., anabolic steroids), their use in the absence of a good training program will lead to some disappointment. In a famous study published in the *New England Journal of Medicine,* one group of subjects was given testosterone only (no exercise) for 10 weeks and saw moderate but inconsistent changes in lean mass. While some subjects did gain between 4 and 9 pounds of lean mass, others gained very little. However, take these same guys, put them on the same dose of steroids *and* on a weight-training program, and they'll consistently gain 13 to 15 pounds of lean mass. See what a difference training makes?

Wait, before you get ahead of yourself, we'd better qualify that last discussion. Don't think for a second that we're recommending the use of steroids here. We're certainly not! This book is about building muscle the natural way. Of course, in all fairness, we do believe that steroids are legitimate medications used for legitimate medical conditions. In times of androgen deficiency (as diagnosed by your doctor), they're a godsend. But in the absence of clinical problems, they shouldn't be considered. And we're not going to drop a load of scare tactics on you. Rather, we say that they shouldn't be considered because the program contained in this book is designed to help you pack on *more* weight than you'd gain by just popping some steroids! Seriously, give us any two scrawny guys, put one on a random training/nutrition program and steroids and the other on this program, and we'll guarantee that the guy on our program will get the best results in the *long term.* Over the short term, 10 to 12 weeks of training, the gains will be similar. But after another 12 weeks, the steroid user will have lost much of his gains, while the guy following our plan will have gotten bigger. Which would you prefer? Twelve weeks of increased muscle mass followed by a steady decline to your previous size, or constant progress?

So that's our stance on steroid use. Sure, lots of people out there are using them. But many of these users are jeopardizing their health for no good reason. If we're giving you the choice between a drug that'll make you big yet may jeopardize your health versus a program that will make you big and improve your health, which are you going to choose?

So if steroids are out of the question, why did we bring them up in the first place? Well, we wanted to illustrate the fact that even with the use of powerful steroids, there still is no magic pill that'll allow you to get the results you're looking for without putting in the required effort. And this is true even more so with supplements. To get bigger, you need to have your training and nutritional programs optimized first. Then, and only then, should you consider supplements such as creatine, workout stimulants, cortisol suppressors, testosterone boosters, etc. We're serious; if your nutrition isn't optimized, your money will be much better spent on food versus supplements. Want an example? Our typical clients come to us frustrated with their gains. After examining their supplement and grocery bills, we often realize why. They're spending money on bricklayers but not bricks (remember this analogy from earlier?). After we reduce their supplement bills, using the supplement money they've saved to buy groceries, they end up making the kind of progress they're looking for. To them, it's an epiphany. To us, it's just good sense (and cents).

But what about those of you who nail down the nutrition and training and are looking for that little extra boost? We'll present a number of supplements available on the market today that have been suggested (by manufacturers) to offer benefit in your quest for brawniness.

You'll notice that we'll review individual nutrients/supplements rather than combination products as they are commonly sold. Research tends to be done on individual ingredients because researchers are interested in single-ingredient studies that advance the state of the scientific literature. On the contrary, supplement companies are more interested in product-specific, patentable formulae that include multiple substances. Although combination products have become very popular, so much so that individual ingredients are becoming increasingly difficult to find, there is often little data to suggest that these combinations offer any additional benefit. While supplement companies would have you believe that their own combinations produce a unique, positive synergy, it is equally likely that their combination could negate the proven beneficial effects of individual ingredients. It's also equally plausible that, worse yet, their chosen combination could produce harmful interactions. For this reason, in this book, we will address only specific ingredients. It's also for this reason that we typically recommend individual ingredients to our clients, including our elite athletes, rather than specific product formulations.

MUSCLE-BUILDING SUPPLEMENTS

For organizational purposes, we've grouped the supplements according to the following categories:

1. Muscle-building supplements

2. Ergogenic (performance-enhancing) aids

3. Recovery/replenishment supplements

We've included supplements that are being sold to improve muscle mass or strength-exercise performance. Below each supplement, we offer a brief description of what it's supposed to do and whether research actually supports its use. We've put an asterisk (*) next to all supplements we consider essential when following our nutrition and training programs. Finally, at the end of the chapter, we'll give you specific instructions for how to use the supplements we consider essential.

Chasteberry

Chasteberry (also called vitex) has recently gained attention as a way to boost the natural production of testosterone in men. Chasteberry contains flavonoids, terpenes, and sterols, all phytochemicals known for drug-like effects. The particular phytochemicals in chasteberry have been suggested to raise testosterone concentrations and therefore build muscle mass and strength. While early investigations suggest that testosterone concentrations may increase modestly in men supplementing with chasteberry, it is not known whether this will translate into improved muscle building or strength. In fact, the small increases seen in testosterone concentrations with some herbal formulae are not typically correlated with improvements in muscle mass unless an individual is hypogonadal (producing too little testosterone naturally).

Conjugated Linoleic Acid (CLA)

CLA is actually a series of uncommon fatty acids, found largely in dairy and beef, which have been shown, principally in animal models, to reduce fat mass. However, CLA has also been shown to have anticatabolic effects, reducing tissue loss after invading organisms (virus or bacteria) or acute trauma (burns, broken bones, etc.) overwhelm the immune system. While the animal data are strongly suggestive of an impressive muscle-building and nutrient-partitioning effect (shifting more of the energy you eat toward muscles rather than fat cells), human data have been less clear. Although still primarily sold for fat reduction, consumers interested in CLA as a muscle-building aid should be aware that very little human data exist and a dramatic effect is unlikely.

Fish Oil*

Fish oil is rich in a specific group of fatty acids (omega-3 fatty acids) that are commonly missing in the North American diet. When added to the diet, these fats (especially the most active DHA and EPA components of omega-3s) have been shown to improve insulin sensitivity in muscle cells while decreasing it in fat cells. As a result, nutrients are more likely to be shunted toward muscle instead of adipose tissue. In addition to improved carbohydrate storage, fish oil may improve the efficiency of protein storage, increase metabolic rate, and increase lean mass. Although this type of fat has profound effects on the body, fish oil is completely safe and actually increases the overall health profile including reducing cardiovascular disease risk, cancer risk, and diabetes risk. Fish oil supplementation is probably essential for exercisers and nonexercisers alike. Everyone should be taking fish oil regardless of their health and fitness priorities.

Myostatin Inhibitors

Myostatin is a protein that negatively regulates muscle growth. At a certain point, myostatin is released to prevent muscle from getting "too big." Interestingly, a specific sulfo-polysaccharide extract (CSP-3) cultured from algae has been discovered, in the laboratory, to bind to the myostatin protein and prevent myostatin from keeping muscles smaller. If this supplement can bind to the myostatin protein in the body, it could neutralize the inhibition that the myostatin protein puts on new muscle growth. However, no one knows whether or not this actually happens. Just because a compound binds to myostatin in a laboratory experiment done outside of the body doesn't mean that it will survive digestion, find the skeletal muscle, make it into the muscle, and bind to the myostatin protein in the muscle. Until more research is done, we suggest skipping this one, especially since myostatin is found in the heart as well as skeletal muscle.

Nitric Oxide Boosters

Nitric oxide (NO) is a free radical gas produced in the body from the breakdown of the amino acid arginine. The primary function of NO is to relax smooth muscle, like the kind in your blood vessels. In doing so, NO can decrease blood pressure, increase bloodflow to muscles and organs, and prevent blood platelets from clumping up (platelet clumping is a bad thing because it can damage vessels). So upon first glance, it looks like NO-boosting supplements might be health promoting. But how can they help build muscle? Well, some supplement companies have suggested that increased bloodflow to muscles might be anabolic (although there is no good evidence that NO-induced bloodflow increases can build muscle). Interestingly, however, NO boosters don't actually contain any nitric oxide. Rather, they contain the amino acid precursors for NO. Whether these amino acids actually raise NO is another question entirely. So, in the end, although some users report a better "pump" when training, there's little evidence that this bestselling supplement actually helps build muscle. And even less evidence that this supplement is actually safe. We suggest saying no to NO for now.

Prohormones

Prohormones come in an increasing number of types with slightly different intended results. These include muscle and/or strength gain, increased aggressiveness during training, improved sexual performance, and cosmetic physique effects. These improvements are expected to occur as a result of increases in testosterone or testosterone precursor concentrations in the blood. At the time of this writing, prohormones are legal. However, by the time this book is printed, the governmental lobby that made these hormones "endangered" may have succeeded in banning them. In our opinion, that's probably a good thing since many of the prohormones don't work, and the ones that do can either lead to increased estrogen concentrations in the blood in addition to the testosterone boost or can lead to suppression of natural testosterone production. Therefore, once you go off, bye-bye gains.

Protein Supplements*

Protein supplements, simply put, provide a convenient way to meet your daily protein goal if you can't find a way to get all of your daily protein from food. In this way, we consider protein supplements more closely related to food than supplements. One way to think of protein supplements is that they are lower-quality alternatives to chicken, beef, fish, etc. We say lower quality because they don't contain the other vitamins and minerals that chicken, beef, fish, etc., contain. Most protein supplements currently available are made of one or more components of milk protein. Whey protein, a popular supplement, makes up about 20 percent of the protein found in milk, while casein protein, a less popular supplement, makes up about 80 percent of the protein found in milk. If you're interested in using a protein supplement during the day, your best bet is to use a whey/casein blend. This is typically listed as "milk protein isolate" or "milk protein blend" on supplement labels. This blend is ideal for meals during the Growth and Recovery Phases of the day because it contains slow- and fast-digesting proteins, fast protein playing a role in improving protein synthesis, and slow protein playing a role in decreasing protein breakdown. As you'll see in the recovery/regeneration section of this chapter, fast proteins are more ideal for nutrition during the Energy and Anabolic Phases because fast proteins are more quickly delivered to muscle.

ERGOGENIC AIDS

Here's a list of several popular supplements proposed to offer a performance enhancing benefit and how they stack up.

Caffeine

Numerous published studies support caffeine's effects as a central nervous system stimulant that increases wakefulness. Large doses (3 to 8 mg/kg body weight) also reliably increase fatty acid release from body storage, which has been suggested as a mechanism for caffeine's ability to increase time-to-exhaustion in endurance activity and spare muscle glycogen. The fat mobilization effects may potentially affect fat reduction in exercisers over time as well. Caffeine also increases metabolic rate about 5 to 10 percent, depending on dose. Weight trainers often use caffeine just before training to increase their wakefulness and strength. While single acute doses before training may help performance, chronic use may negatively impact glucose tolerance. So one dose before training is okay. One dose every hour is not.

Carbohydrate/Sports Drinks

Carbohydrates are taken up by exercising muscles and used for fuel. Post exercise, they hasten glycogen replenishment. Fluids can also help keep a body hydrated and keep body temperature in the comfort zone. This means the prevention of performance-killing dehydration. Numerous published studies have demonstrated the benefits of carbohydrate beverages on physical performance—particularly with events over an hour in duration. They are also well documented to enhance recovery from muscle-depleting exercise—both aerobic and anaerobic. While these types of drinks can also provide energy during strength exercise, as discussed in the previous chapter, the addition of protein and certain amino acids makes these drinks more effective for weight trainers.

Creatine*

Creatine monohydrate ingestion increases skeletal muscle free creatine and phosphocreatine concentrations, the naturally occurring energy pools that replenish ATP (cell energy) directly. This uptake also draws water into the cell, causing the muscle to swell. This means better anaerobic power and muscle strength. This cell swelling causes a rapid increase in muscle mass (mostly increases in water content). However, in the long run, this may also increase skeletal muscle protein synthesis and muscle glycogen storage. Since creatine monohydrate in powdered form is the only research-supported form of creatine, that's what we recommend. Also, despite anecdotal reports, no side effects other than mild gastric distress (which subsides) have been validated in the scientific literature. While about 80 percent of creatine users see the aforementioned benefits, 20 percent have been considered "nonresponders." Some believe that these "nonresponders" don't respond because they already may have high dietary intakes of creatine from whole foods. Finally, we don't believe that a "loading phase" is necessary. Rather, taking a few grams each day is probably the best way to use creatine monohydrate.

Ribose

The sugar ribose is a precursor to adenosine (the A in ATP). As the theory goes, by increasing the amount of ribose available in the cells, cellular energy might be improved, leading to improvements in performance. Unfortunately, research hasn't supported this idea, and ribose supplementation might not offer the benefits scientists originally thought it would. Since ribose may function similarly to creatine, it's probably better to just take the creatine.

Tyrosine

The body converts large multigram doses of tyrosine into the catecholamines (fight or flight hormones) epinephrine and norepinephrine. Published research indicates that tyrosine can improve reaction time and attention, reduce the perception of stress and the stress hormone response, and can actually improve weight-lifting performance. This category of ergogenic aids (neurotransmitter formulas) is becoming popular as scientists learn more about the effects of various neurotransmitters on central nervous system function as it relates to exercise. In athletes, the increased attention, reduction in performance drop-off during sustained efforts, the reduced reaction time, and the blunted stress response are all of benefit. The recreational exerciser, however, may not see great benefit from tyrosine, because training might not be frequent or intense enough. Tyrosine should probably be used on an empty stomach before training or later in the day between meals.

RECOVERY SUPPLEMENTS

Here's a list of several popular supplements proposed to offer recovery benefits and how they stack up.

Beta-Sitosterols

Plant sterols have been shown to possess anti-inflammatory properties and immune-modulating properties and may affect the anabolic to catabolic hormone ratio. Studies have shown that a combination of beta-sitosterol and beta-sitosterol glucoside can help prevent the damage normally seen during marathon training and competition. This means improved immune function and better recovery. Beta-sitosterols are present in most plants, fruits, and vegetables and are structurally similar to cholesterol. However, you can't get enough in the diet because they are bound to plant fibers and are often difficult to digest and absorb. That is why supplemental plant sterols are necessary to achieve the positive results described above. While these aren't necessary every day, they may help immune function and recovery during intense periods of training or if you're chronically getting sick.

Branched Chain Amino Acids*

As discussed in Chapter 15, the BCAA (especially leucine) have been shown to increase skeletal muscle protein synthesis during the postexercise period, a critical period for promoting muscle recovery. In addition, the presence of BCAA in a carbohydrate drink can boost the insulin response, potentially increasing muscle glycogen storage. Since the BCAA are particularly effective in correcting the negative protein status associated with the postexercise period, causing a shift from muscle catabolism to muscle anabolism, they're a staple during the Energy and Anabolic Phases. Just don't go overboard. Since amino acids compete for absorption, BCAA may compete with other amino acids for entry into the body if too many are consumed relative to the other amino acids.

Glutamine*

Although glutamine is usually made in sufficient quantities in the body, during times of stress (such as injury and infection), the body may fall short. This amino acid is used in the gastrointestinal tract, immune cells, and skeletal muscle and therefore, if the body falls short in its glutamine production, these cells may compete for glutamine use, potentially weakening GI function and immune function and causing a catabolic state. While glutamine supplementation can help injured patients and help boost immune function, it is unlikely that glutamine will actually cause direct performance benefits and/or increases in muscle mass. However, when added to a protein and carbohydrate beverage, glutamine causes a larger insulin response, potentially leading to more glycogen or muscle protein recovery.

L-Carnitine L-Tartrate

During high-intensity exercise, carnitine concentrations in the blood and muscle are reduced. In blood vessels, this depletion could lead to compromised bloodflow and poor oxygen delivery. Carnitine supplementation may prevent this compromise in bloodflow, allowing more tissue perfusion, more oxygen delivery, and less muscle damage. Specifically, studies have shown that L-carnitine L-tartrate can reduce muscle disruption and markers of muscle breakdown after exercise as well as attenuate the rise in markers of oxidative damage. Despite past research that had not been positive, L-carnitine supplements have remained popular. Since previous research examined only a narrow hypothesis (that carnitine could increase fatty acid transport into the mitochondrion, leading to increased aerobic performance and increased fat burning), and results were scattered and far from definitive, many athletes and nutritionists have written off this popular dietary supplement. However, new data have begun to offer some support for its popular use in recovery.

Whey Protein*

Whey protein promotes a rapid rise in blood amino acid concentrations, rapidly delivering these amino acids to skeletal muscle to promote recovery of muscle protein status. Whey makes up 20 percent of the protein found in milk and is the rapidly digested portion of milk. After ingestion of some types of whey protein, blood amino acid concentrations rise within 15 minutes, as does muscle protein synthesis. As with BCAA, when whey protein is coadministered with carbohydrates, there is a synergistic insulin release, promoting rapid carbohydrate storage. As a result, whey protein (especially hydrolyzed whey protein) is an excellent protein choice for the workout and postworkout periods (the Energy and Anabolic Phases) due to its fast digestion and absorption. Slower proteins are desirable for the remainder of the day (the Growth and Recovery Phases).

Phosphatidylserine

Often weight trainers and coaches consider only the "gym" stressors as the most significant in the recovery process. However, other life stressors can be as important as or even more important than what's happening during your hour in the gym. When job, family, house, and financial pressures mount, the hormone cortisol might be working overtime, putting a serious damper on your recovery and even causing extra fat accumulation around your midsection. Phosphatidylserine is a phospholipid that has been shown to reduce cortisol concentrations in the blood. Although this isn't a staple, when our athletes are about to begin intense training periods, they typically use this compound once or twice per day to buffer their combined training and lifestyle stressors.

Recovery Drinks*

As discussed in the previous chapter, recovery drinks containing carbohydrate and protein in a 2:1 ratio as well as additional amino acids such as the BCAA, glutamine, and phenylalanine, can, when ingested during the Energy and Anabolic Phases, lead to increased protein synthesis, decreased protein breakdown, increased glycogen resynthesis, and a better anabolic to catabolic hormone ratio. Although making your own drink with whey protein, amino acids, and carbohydrate can be as effective as (and potentially less expensive than) commercial recovery drinks, these drinks make it easy to get the right macronutrients in the right proportions. So if you don't want to make your own home blend, pick one of these up.

We'll admit it: Making sense of supplementation can be confusing at times. Supplement manufacturers are constantly bombarding the magazines (and you) with pseudoscientific ads promoting the quality and effectiveness of their products. And make no mistake about it; the people hired to

SUPPLEMENT USE AND TIMING

PHASE	SUPPLEMENTS
Energy	Sip carbohydrate/protein (recovery) drink prior to and during training. This drink should contain 0.8 g/kg carbohydrate, 0.4 g/kg protein, 3–5 g BCAA, 3 g glutamine, and 3 g phenylalanine
Anabolic	Drink carbohydrate/protein (recovery) drink immediately after training. This drink should contain 0.8 g/kg carbohydrate, 0.4 g/kg protein, 3–5 g BCAA, 3 g glutamine, and 3 g phenylalanine. Add to this drink 3–5 g creatine
Growth	During this phase, most meals should be solid food but can contain milk protein isolates (whey/casein), if you need something convenient. Furthermore, fish oil should be included during this phase (see menu plan for how much)
Recovery	During this phase, most meals should be solid food but can contain milk protein isolates (whey/casein), if you need something convenient. Furthermore, fish oil should be included during this phase (see menu plan for how much)

"hook" you are good at what they do. So with all of these supplement ads and choices out there, it's easy to simply curl up into the fetal position and give up. But there's no need for frustration. It's all a matter of perspective. Although there are new supplements, many without research testing, being launched all the time, you're probably not missing out on much if you just sit back and wait until some research is done before trying them. In this chapter, we've listed a number of the most popular ones out there today and have highlighted the essentials that will undoubtedly help you in your efforts to put some muscle on those bones. Use these in conjunction with the training and nutritional plan contained herein, and you're guaranteed the fast track to results.

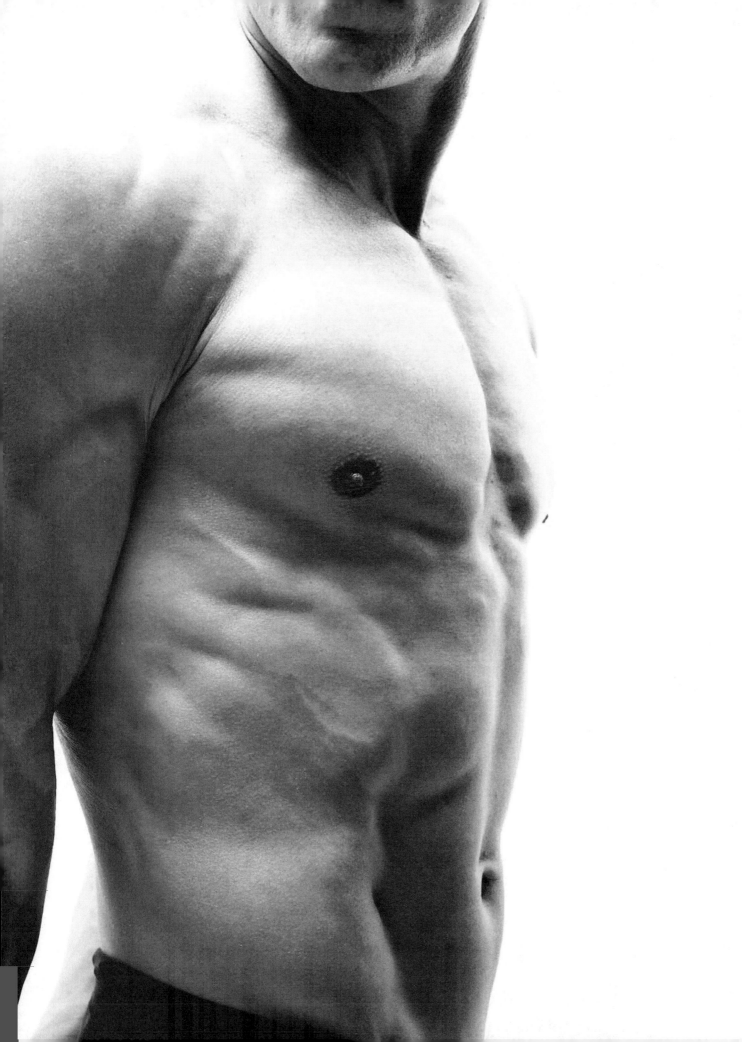

BECOMING A
NUTRITIONAL BOY SCOUT

》》The motto of the Boy Scouts and of this chapter is "Be prepared." Prepared for what? Be prepared for anything and everything that might stand in the way of your progress. As we've discussed earlier, it's going to be challenging to apply all of the nutrition strategies laid out in this book including eating enough total energy, employing the principles of nutrient timing, following good post-exercise nutritional strategies, etc. Putting together a plan is nothing. Changing your habits so that you adhere closely to the plan is something else altogether. Remember, it's not that it's difficult. It's just that most people overestimate how hard it will be and underestimate how long it will take. However, with any degree of commitment, you'll be a Jedi nutritional master in no time. As master Yoda says, "Try? There is no try; there is only do and do not."

In order to put you on the right track to nutritional knighthood, in this chapter, we present a series of effective strategies, including the Breakfast Ritual, strategies for snacking at work, and strategies for eating lunch on the go. Furthermore, we'll present strategies for emergency situations that defy planning. For example, what happens if you get called to an unforeseen business meeting when you should be heading down to TGIFriday's for your daily lunch of two lean burgers (no bun, please) and an extra-large garden salad? And what happens if you get called into work unexpectedly and haven't planned your meals? How about if you sleep in, get stuck in traffic, or have an unexpectedly late Saturday night with your date? What will you do when "life" seems to get in the way of eating properly?

Do you currently have strategies for getting in your meals under these conditions? If not, you'd better develop some. As we mentioned earlier, the secret to success in bulking up (or getting lean, for that matter) isn't novelty. No special program, special supplement, or special meal plan (that you follow only 50 percent of the time) will swoop in to give you the gains you seek unless you follow it regularly. Consistency is the secret to uncommon results. And consistency knows that life is bound to get in the way, so it plans for obstacles and finds alternate routes around them.

So let's discuss how to get consistent by looking at the sample meal plan presented in Chapter 13.

In looking at this plan, it should be obvious that you'll need some serious strategies for preparing these meals each training day. After all, a few solid meals will have to be eaten at work, and they're not necessarily going to be cooking themselves, are they?

So up out of your chair; it's time for another store run right now. That's right, we're getting bossy again. Without some food preparation and storage support systems, you'll be fumbling around your kitchen until you finally consider your efforts an exercise in futility and go back to your old, scrawny ways. Remember the First Supper. You're eating like a big guy now, so to keep up the good work, we want you to head to the store right away, and pick up the items listed below. We promise they'll make your nutritional life much, much easier.

)) One countertop grill. Make sure to get one with a large surface area because this makes cooking all your lean beef and chicken sausage for the day a simple, 10-minute process.

)) Five large plastic or glass rectangular containers. These containers should be airtight and will be used to store anything from cooked quinoa and yams to cut fruits and vegetables in your refrigerator. One suc-

4,600-KCAL MENU FOR THE HYPERTROPHY-CHALLENGED

MEAL #1
12 egg whites

1 slice regular cheese

Chopped fresh veggies

1 tablespoon flax oil

2 fish oil capsules

1 cup green tea

MEAL #2
1 cup organic yogurt

1 scoop protein powder

2 fish oil capsules

MEAL #3
2 chicken sausage links

Organic spinach

1 cup organic carrots

2 tablespoons apple-cider vinegar

1 tablespoon flax oil

4 fish oil capsules

MEAL #4 PRE-WORKOUT
1 serving recovery drink

MEAL #5 DURING WORKOUT
1 serving recovery drink

MEAL #6 IMMEDIATELY AFTER WORKOUT
1 serving recovery drink

MEAL #7
1 cup yogurt

1 scoop protein powder

1 or 2 pieces fruit

2½ cups cereal

MEAL #8
4 oz. lean beef

Organic spinach

1 cup organic carrots

2 tablespoons apple-cider vinegar

½ cup quinoa (or yam)

1 piece fruit

MEAL #9
4 oz. lean beef

Organic spinach

1 cup organic carrots

2 tablespoons apple-cider vinegar

1 tablespoon olive oil

2 fish oil capsules

¼ cup cashews

cessful preparation strategy is to cook some of your food for the week on Sunday night so that you can easily spoon it out when it's time to eat each day. Also, you can precut your fruit and veggies and spoon them out when it's time to eat them or package them up for the day.

>> **Five small plastic or glass square containers.** These containers should also be airtight and will be used to carry all of your meals with you each day. You're going to want to package all your meals unless you absolutely know that you'll be eating elsewhere. This way if you get stuck in an unexpected situation, you'll have food nearby and won't have to miss a meal or make a poor food choice (i.e., vending machine or fast-food joint).

>> **Four plastic or glass shaker bottles.** These shakers should be 1 liter in volume and have a good screw-on top to prevent leaking. You can put your powders for the day in these bottles, and add water when needed.

>> **One cooler/lunch box.** Your cooler/lunch box should have enough room to store all of your meals for the day including your three or four shaker bottles. Keep this cooler nearby so that you'll have access to your food whenever it's time to eat.

>> **One watch with alarm.** If you don't already have one, a watch with a timer is critical for the initial stages of your program. Set your watch to the specific times of the day when you need to eat.

Once you have these items, you're ready to perform the Breakfast Ritual. If you follow our instruction, you should be able to cook all your food for the day in 30 minutes or less. That's right, all 4,600 kcal can be cooked and packaged in 30 minutes or less. Once all the meals are done, all you've gotta do is sit down, eat your breakfast, and take off for the day. Alternatively, if you don't want to wake up earlier than you already do, simply cook your meals as described below before you go to bed at night.

THE BREAKFAST (OR EVENING) RITUAL

1. Begin to boil water for tea, and plug in your countertop grill.

2. Place a skillet on a heating element, spray the skillet with cooking spray, and pour in the egg whites and chopped fresh veggies.

3. While these are cooking, throw two 8-ounce burgers and two sausage links on the grill.

4. While everything is cooking, open three rectangular containers, and make your three spinach and carrot salads (one salad gets ¼ cup of cashews and the other a piece of fruit, which can be precut.)

5. At this point, flip the omelet, and place one piece of cheese on top.

6. The water should be boiling, so pour your tea.

7. Place a serving of recovery drink powder in each of three shaker bottles, and screw on the lids (no water until necessary).

8. Put 1 cup yogurt in each of two additional square containers; add in 1 scoop of protein powder, and mix.

9. Take burgers and chicken sausages off the heating element, and place each serving in a square container.

10. Place ½ cup quinoa or 1 yam in an additional rectangular container.

11. Place 2½ cups cereal in a plastic re-sealable bag.

12. At this point, place the square containers, rectangular containers, shaker bottles, and plastic resealable bag in your cooler with a bottle of flax oil, a bottle of fish oil, a bottle of apple cider vinegar, and one or two pieces of fruit. Throw in a couple of condiments as well, such as pesto, mustard, and so on.

With the breakfast (or nighttime) ritual completed, you can sit down to enjoy your breakfast knowing you're nutritionally prepared for the long day ahead. Find a microwave oven at work or school, and you can heat up each meal when it's time to eat it.

Of course, the full breakfast ritual might not suit your particular lifestyle. After all, some of you might eat lunch and dinner at restaurants each day. If so, you'll have to find suitable substitutes for two of the meals in the plan. If it's a P + F meal, you can choose meat, salads, and side orders of veggies. (Remember to bring your fish oil as well as a little container of flax oil and vinegar to add to your salad.) If it's a P + C meal, you can choose very lean meats, salads, and veggies, fruit, and good grain sources. But just be sure that you can actually make it to the restaurant. If you think there's a chance of missing your lunch or dinner due to working late or emergency meetings, it's important that you package up a few meals before you leave for the day. If you don't get to eat the meal because you got to the restaurant after all, just save it for another day.

Others of you might not eat out every day but may leave for work knowing that two or three of your daily meals can be eaten at night when you're already home. Perhaps you do the cooking, or your significant other does. Either way, you don't want to lug around a few extra meals each day if you don't have to. In this situation, simply cook the meals you need for the day in the morning, and wait till you get home to prepare the rest.

And others of you might simply dislike food preparation so much, yet not have the time to eat at restaurants daily. In this case, you might entertain hiring a food preparation service. It's likely that there will be such a service in your immediate area, and if you live in a major city, there will likely be many to choose from. These types of food service companies will deliver hot lunches and dinners made to your specifications for a daily fee. However, since they probably don't offer much in the way of protein powders, you'll still have to prepare some of the easy meals for yourself. The others you can leave up to the pros.

With these basic preparation strategies laid out, here are a few additional strategies our clients have found useful when the unexpected happens:

Have Cooler, Will Travel

Always have some type of food with you so that you can eat "in a pinch." Bad food decisions are made out of hunger, and hunger comes when you've forgotten to eat and/or don't have meals with you. Fill up that cooler of yours with the good foods you'll need to eat to get bigger, and lug it around wherever you go. Then you will never have any excuses for not packing on the mass.

On the Seventh Day, He Cooked

While five of nine meals on the plan laid out so far will take you virtually no time to prepare (three of them involve putting powder in a shaker bottle, and two involve spooning out some yogurt and powder into a bowl and mixing), the other meals may take a bit longer. One way to expedite this process is to shop on Saturday or Sunday, and grill your meat selections for the week (chicken sausages and burgers in this example). If you cook up a bunch of yams and/or quinoa as well as chopping up your veggies and fruits for the week, the Breakfast Ritual is significantly easier. Store these prepared foods in your large rectangular containers, and all you'll need to do is spoon out these foods each morning. (In order to prevent the browning that occurs when the cut fruit is exposed to the air, dip the cut fruit in a little lemon juice.)

90 Percent Is Still an "A"

Once in a while, you'll find it very difficult to get all your meals prepared as suggested. Sometimes you'll accidentally run out of groceries. Other times, you'll miss your alarm clock and wake up late for work. Other times, you'll forget your cooler on the roof of the car, and it'll be but a distant memory by the time you get to work. On these days, do your best. Don't throw up your hands in the air and revert to old habits. Rather, try to eat as closely to the meal plan as possible. Besides, perfection isn't a requisite for success on this plan. Rather, we typically suggest following the plan with 90 percent accuracy. This means that you can probably get away with not following the plan 10 percent of the time. Translated into actual meals, since you'll be eating about 51 meals per week, the 90 percent rule dictates that at least 46 of them should be "perfect," and you've got room for five "cheat meals."

Excuse Me, Waitress

When you choose to eat out at restaurants, in order to ensure that you're getting the best nutrition possible, you need to be specific about what you want. Ordering items on the menu might be a mistake because the protein portions are often small and covered in undesirable sauces. Rather than simply picking a menu item and chancing that it'll be good for you, order something specific to your goals. If your plan calls for a P + C meal, order your protein source, a steamed vegetable source, a large salad, and something like a baked potato or some rice. Don't be afraid to ask how much meat you get, and if necessary, double it. Also get your dressings on the side, or better yet, get the salad with no dressing, and bring your own with you in a small container. Remember, you're leaving the waitress a tip, so be sure that she earns it. Make sure you know exactly what you are ordering, and don't be afraid to ask for something specific.

Is That a Protein Bar in Your Pocket?

Don't go longer than 3 hours without eating. On any given day, if you know that you will have some serious nutrition challenges and simply can't get all the food prepared, stock that cooler with quick snacks from the list below:

» Beef, turkey, or ostrich jerky/ pepperettes

» Mixed nuts

» Fruit

» Part-skim cheese sticks

» Protein shakes, made with a high-quality milk protein blend, yogurt, olive/flax oil

» Protein bars (choose a high-protein/high-fiber variety)

Although a cooler full of these isn't necessarily optimal for day-to-day nutrition, if you're on a road trip or can't get access to your normal meals, they're a good substitute.

Of course, these are just a few ideas to help you make like a Boy Scout and "be prepared." Remember, the difference between those who are in shape and those who "should get in shape" is as simple as duplicating success. We've created the success plan; now it's your turn to duplicate it.

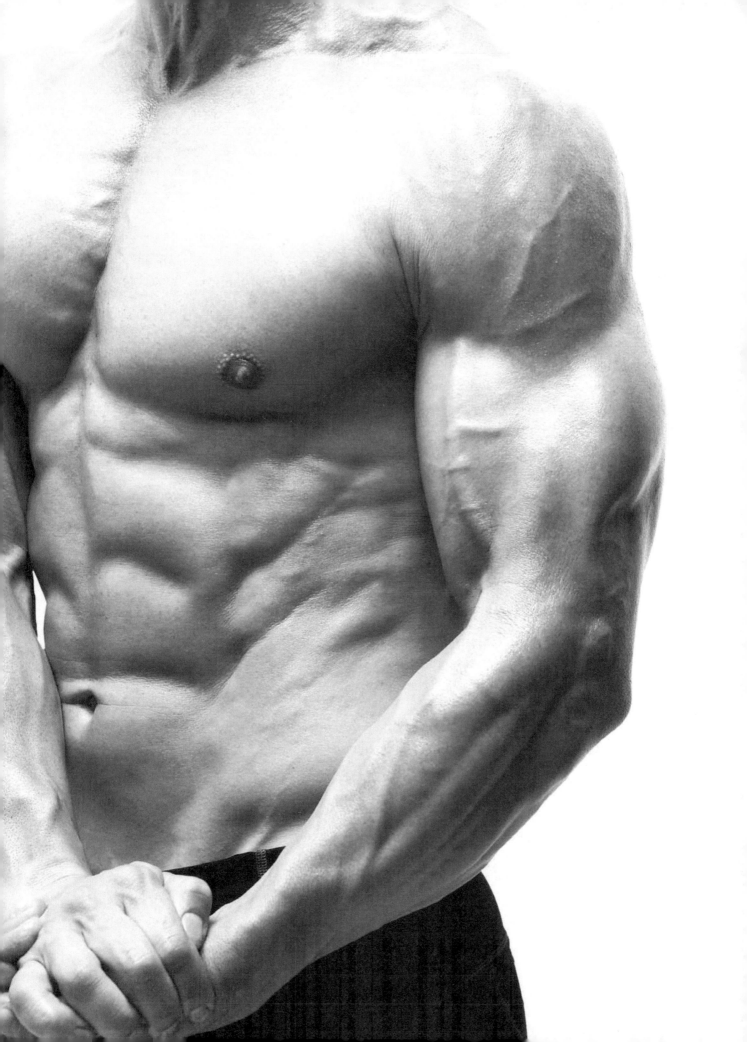

18

EAT THIS!

>> Now that we've addressed the principles of creating an optimal meal plan, given you strategies for adapting your plan, and offered strategies for consistently following your plan, we'd like to give you an example of these principles in action. While we will present four meal plans, one for each phase, remember, these aren't necessarily optimal for you. Rather, they are templates you should work from using the results of your own calorie calculations (Chapter 13), the time of day you train (Chapter 14), and your own outcome-based response to adjust appropriately.

In the following examples, we've created weekly nutrition plans for a reference male who is 5'7" tall, 154 pounds, and 10 percent body fat, and who trains in the afternoon. (We know, most scrawny, ectomorphic, hypertrophy-challenged types are tall and lanky, and our reference male is only 5'7", but remember, this guy is just an example of the physical reference point most researchers use as a starting point). In this plan, the energy intake increases as appropriate throughout the 15-week program. However, the program in this chapter is just an example. To create your most effective program, employ the strategies outlined in Chapter 13 by plugging your own numbers into the equations and determining your own energy needs. Then, using the biweekly, outcome-based strategy presented in the Decision-Making Matrix (page 182), you can optimize.

To refresh your memory, this strategy entails assessing your progress objectively (i.e., making regular body weight and body fat measurements) and using this assessment to determine whether you need more calories or not. If you're not making the appropriate progress, you'll need to alter your energy intake by about 250 kcal until you start seeing movement in the positive direction. We typically recommend making these changes every 2 weeks.

In looking over the meal plans presented here, you'll notice that the menu is relatively similar throughout. We do this for a reason. We want you to begin to build regular eating habits before you change things around drastically. However, with this said, we built in variety. For example, rather than recommending a specific type of meat, we suggest you choose from a variety of options including extra-lean ground beef, sirloin steak, chicken breast, extra-lean ground chicken breast, extra-lean ground turkey breast, turkey breast, turkey or chicken sausage, fresh fish (salmon, cod, tuna, etc.), canned tuna, and so on. Also, we don't recommend specific fruit selections; rather, we recommend you choose from a variety of options including 1 medium-size apple, pear, orange, or banana, ½ cup berries, or ¼ cup dried fruit. You are also free to include a diversity of vegetables in your salad mixes.

Sure, to most individuals changing their dietary strategies for the better, even this wide variety of options seems somehow restrictive. But if you think about it, assuming you choose a variety of fruits, meats, and veggies, this meal plan provides a diversity of foods that most North Americans wouldn't get even in a full week! So before you complain about "having to eat the same things every day," first examine whether this is actually true or not. Ask yourself whether you're actually getting less variety or if you're just getting less variety of crappy foods. If you find yourself becoming "bored," perhaps your real complaint is that you don't like eliminating the garbage foods you had been eating regularly. If this is your complaint, it's a common one. No one does like it at first. But once the muscle starts packing on your frame, and once your palate adjusts to the new selections (and trust us, it will), you'll be happy you decided to hang in there through the boredom. And remember the 90 percent rule. You've still got 10 percent of the week to eat some foods not on the menu.

MENU #1—PHASE I: THE CORRECTIVE PHASE (VARIABLE LENGTH)

EXAMPLE CLIENT:

Client Height: 5'7"; Client Weight: 154 pounds; Client Fat Percent: 10 percent

Nutrition for Training Days (3 times per week)

›› First Breakfast Meal

ITEM	CALORIES	PROTEIN	%	CARBS	%	FAT	%
250 ml egg white	108.0	25.0	93	2.0	7	0.0	0
2 whole omega-3 eggs	137.0	13.0	38	1.0	3	9.0	59
1/4 cup mixed beans (kidney, etc.)	52.0	3.0	23	10.0	77	0.0	0
1 cup mixed vegetables	44.0	1.0	9	10.0	91	0.0	0
25 grams cashews	160.0	6.0	15	7.0	18	12.0	68
2 fish oil capsules	18.0	0.0	0	0.0	0	2.0	100
TOTAL	519.0	48.0	37	30.0	23	23.0	40

›› Second Breakfast Meal

ITEM	CALORIES	PROTEIN	%	CARBS	%	FAT	%
400 grams plain yogurt	249.0	14.0	22	19.0	31	13.0	47
25 grams almonds	161.0	6.0	15	5.0	12	13.0	73
1 scoop milk protein blend	106.0	20.0	75	2.0	8	2.0	17
TOTAL	516.0	40.0	31	26.0	20	28.0	49

›› First Lunch Meal

ITEM	CALORIES	PROTEIN	%	CARBS	%	FAT	%
200 grams lean meat (raw weight)	155.1	34.6	89	0.0	0	1.9	11
Large garden salad	65.0	4.0	25	10.0	62	1.0	14
1 teaspoon flax oil	45.0	0.0	0	0.0	0	5.0	100
1 teaspoon olive oil	45.0	0.0	0	0.0	0	5.0	100
50 grams cheese	126.0	6.0	19	12.0	38	6.0	43
2 fish oil capsules	18.0	0.0	0	0.0	0	2.0	100
TOTAL	454.1	44.6	39	22.0	19	20.9	41

›› Second Lunch Meal

ITEM	CALORIES	PROTEIN	%	CARBS	%	FAT	%
200 grams lean meat (raw weight)	155.1	34.6	89	0.0	0	1.9	11
Large garden salad	65.0	4.0	25	10.0	62	1.0	14
1 teaspoon flax oil	45.0	0.0	0	0.0	0	5.0	100
1 teaspoon olive oil	45.0	0.0	0	0.0	0	5.0	100
25 grams walnuts	176	4.0	9	4.0	9	16.0	82
TOTAL	486.1	42.6	35	14.0	12	28.9	53

MENU #1—*Continued*

)) *Immediately before Workout*

ITEM	CALORIES	PROTEIN	%	CARBS	%	FAT	%
1 serving recovery drink	336.0	28.0	33	56.0	67	0.0	0
with BCAA, Phe, Glu	0.0	0.0	0	0.0	0	0.0	0
TOTAL	336.0	28.0	33	56.0	67	0.0	0

)) *Sip during Workout*

	CALORIES	PROTEIN	%	CARBS	%	FAT	%
1 serving recovery drink	336.0	28.0	33	56.0	67	0.0	0
with BCAA, Phe, Glu	0.0	0.0	0	0.0	0	0.0	0
TOTAL	336.0	28.0	33	56.0	67	0.0	0

)) *Immediately after Workout*

	CALORIES	PROTEIN	%	CARBS	%	FAT	%
1 serving recovery drink	336.0	28.0	33	56.0	67	0.0	0
with BCAA, Phe, Glu, creatine	0.0	0.0	0	0.0	0	0.0	0
TOTAL	336.0	28.0	33	56.0	67	0.0	0

)) *Second Meal after Workout*

	CALORIES	PROTEIN	%	CARBS	%	FAT	%
200 grams lean meat (raw weight)	155.1	34.6	89	0.0	0	1.9	11
Large garden salad	65.0	4.0	25	10.0	62	1.0	14
1 serving fruit	93.0	1.0	4	20.0	86	1.0	10
50 grams wild rice (raw)	193.0	8.0	17	38.0	79	1.0	5
2 fish oil capsules	18.0	0.0	0	0.0	0	2.0	100
TOTAL	524.1	47.6	36	68.0	52	6.9	12

)) *Pre-Bed Meal*

	CALORIES	PROTEIN	%	CARBS	%	FAT	%
250 ml egg white	108.0	25.0	93	2.0	7	0.0	0
1 serving fruit	93.0	1.0	4	20.0	86	1.0	10
50 grams oats (raw)	187.0	8.0	17	32.0	68	3.0	14
TOTAL	201.0	34.0	68	54.0	107	4.0	18
GRAND TOTAL	3708.4	340.8	37	382.0	41	111.6	27

Note: Weight given is in raw quantities for food (meat, rice, oats) that is to be cooked.

Nutrition for Nontraining Days (4 times per week)

» First Breakfast Meal

ITEM	CALORIES	PROTEIN	%	CARBS	%	FAT	%
250 ml egg white	108.0	25.0	93	2.0	7	0.0	0
2 whole omega-3 eggs	137.0	13.0	38	1.0	3	9.0	59
1/4 cup mixed beans (kidney, etc.)	52.0	3.0	23	10.0	77	0.0	0
1 cup mixed vegetables	44.0	1.0	9	10.0	91	0.0	0
25 grams cashews	160.0	6.0	15	7.0	18	12.0	68
2 fish oil capsules	18.0	0.0	0	0.0	0	2.0	100
TOTAL	519.0	48.0	37	30.0	23	23.0	40

» Second Breakfast Meal

ITEM	CALORIES	PROTEIN	%	CARBS	%	FAT	%
400 grams plain yogurt	249.0	14.0	22	19.0	31	13.0	47
25 grams almonds	161.0	6.0	15	5.0	12	13.0	73
1 scoop milk protein blend	106.0	20.0	75	2.0	8	2.0	17
TOTAL	516.0	40.0	31	26.0	20	28.0	49

» First Lunch Meal

ITEM	CALORIES	PROTEIN	%	CARBS	%	FAT	%
200 grams lean meat (raw weight)	155.1	34.6	89	0.0	0	1.9	11
Large garden salad	65.0	4.0	25	10.0	62	1.0	14
1 teaspoon flax oil	45.0	0.0	0	0.0	0	5.0	100
1 teaspoon olive oil	45.0	0.0	0	0.0	0	5.0	100
50 grams cheese	126.0	6.0	19	12.0	38	6.0	43
2 fish oil capsules	18.0	0.0	0	0.0	0	2.0	100
TOTAL	454.1	44.6	39	22.0	19	20.9	41

» Second Lunch Meal

ITEM	CALORIES	PROTEIN	%	CARBS	%	FAT	%
200 grams lean meat (raw weight)	155.1	34.6	89	0.0	0	1.9	11
Large garden salad	65.0	4.0	25	10.0	62	1.0	14
1 teaspoon flax oil	45.0	0.0	0	0.0	0	5.0	100
1 teaspoon olive oil	45.0	0.0	0	0.0	0	5.0	100
25 grams walnuts	176	4.0	9	4.0	9	16.0	82
TOTAL	486.1	42.6	35	14.0	12	28.9	53

MENU #1—*Continued*

)) *Dinner Meal*

ITEM	CALORIES	PROTEIN	%	CARBS	%	FAT	%
200 grams lean meat (raw weight)	155.1	34.6	89	0.0	0	1.9	11
Large garden salad	65.0	4.0	25	10.0	62	1.0	14
1 serving fruit	93.0	1.0	4	20.0	86	1.0	10
25 grams cashews	329.0	12.0	15	14.0	17	25.0	68
2 fish oil capsules	18.0	0.0	0	0.0	0	2.0	100
TOTAL	660.1	51.6	31	44.0	27	30.9	42

)) *Pre-Bed Meal*

ITEM	CALORIES	PROTEIN	%	CARBS	%	FAT	%
250 ml egg white	108.0	25.0	93	2.0	7	0.0	0
2 whole omega-3 eggs	137.0	13.0	38	1.0	3	9.0	59
1 serving fruit	93.0	1.0	4	20.0	86	1.0	10
50 grams cheese	126.0	6.0	19	12.0	38	6.0	43
TOTAL	338.0	45.0	53	35.0	41	16.0	43
GRAND TOTAL	2973.4	271.8	37	171.0	23	147.6	45

Because we want to gradually ramp up your calories, each week the menu above should be altered as follows:

Week 1: As listed above

Week 2: Add 1 additional scoop protein powder and an additional 25 grams almonds to second breakfast meal.

Week 3: Add 25 grams cashews to first breakfast meal and 25 grams walnuts to second lunch meal.

Since this phase is of variable length based on your own needs, the 3-week ramping strategy might not be optimal for you. Regardless of how long this phase is, however, by the next phase, we want you eating more energy as suggested here.

MENU #2 — PHASE II: THE 5 × 5 PHASE

As a result of the gradually increasing intake in the previous phase, the overall metabolic rate will have increased. In addition, there should have been weight gain (5 to 9 pounds). As a result, this phase will begin with a greater energy requirement than the beginning of the last phase.

Nutrition for Training Days (3 times per week):

❱❱ First Breakfast Meal

ITEM	CALORIES	PROTEIN	%	CARBS	%	FAT	%
250 ml egg white	108.0	25.0	93	2.0	7	0.0	0
2 whole omega-3 eggs	137.0	13.0	38	1.0	3	9.0	59
1/4 cup mixed beans (kidney, etc.)	52.0	3.0	23	10.0	77	0.0	0
1 cup mixed vegetables	44.0	1.0	9	10.0	91	0.0	0
50 grams cashews	320.0	12.0	15	14.0	18	24.0	68
2 fish oil capsules	18.0	0.0	0	0.0	0	2.0	100
TOTAL	679.0	54.0	32	37.0	22	35.0	46

❱❱ Second Breakfast Meal

ITEM	CALORIES	PROTEIN	%	CARBS	%	FAT	%
400 grams plain yogurt	249.0	14.0	22	19.0	31	13.0	47
50 grams almonds	322.0	12.0	15	10.0	12	26.0	73
2 scoops milk protein blend	212.0	40.0	75	4.0	8	4.0	17
TOTAL	783.0	66.0	34	33.0	17	43.0	49

❱❱ First Lunch Meal

ITEM	CALORIES	PROTEIN	%	CARBS	%	FAT	%
200 grams lean meat (raw weight)	155.1	34.6	89	0.0	0	1.9	11
Large garden salad	65.0	4.0	25	10.0	62	1.0	14
1 teaspoon flax oil	45.0	0.0	0	0.0	0	5.0	100
1 teaspoon olive oil	45.0	0.0	0	0.0	0	5.0	100
50 grams cheese	126.0	6.0	19	12.0	38	6.0	43
2 fish oil capsules	18.0	0.0	0	0.0	0	2.0	100
TOTAL	454.1	44.6	39	22.0	19	20.9	41

❱❱ Second Lunch Meal

ITEM	CALORIES	PROTEIN	%	CARBS	%	FAT	%
200 grams lean meat (raw weight)	155.1	34.6	89	0.0	0	1.9	11
Large garden salad	65.0	4.0	25	10.0	62	1.0	14
1 teaspoon flax oil	45.0	0.0	0	0.0	0	5.0	100
1 teaspoon olive oil	45.0	0.0	0	0.0	0	5.0	100
50 grams walnuts	176	4.0	9	4.0	9	16.0	82
TOTAL	486.1	42.6	35	14.0	12	28.9	53

MENU #2—*Continued*

)) *Immediately before Workout*

ITEM	CALORIES	PROTEIN	%	CARBS	%	FAT	%
1 serving recovery drink	336.0	28.0	33	56.0	67	0.0	0
with BCAA, Phe, Glu	0.0	0.0	0	0.0	0	0.0	0
TOTAL	336.0	28.0	33	56.0	67	0.0	0

)) *Sip during Workout*

	CALORIES	PROTEIN	%	CARBS	%	FAT	%
1 serving recovery drink	336.0	28.0	33	56.0	67	0.0	0
with BCAA, Phe, Glu	0.0	0.0	0	0.0	0	0.0	0
TOTAL	336.0	28.0	33	56.0	67	0.0	0

)) *Immediately after Workout*

	CALORIES	PROTEIN	%	CARBS	%	FAT	%
1 serving recovery drink	336.0	28.0	33	56.0	67	0.0	0
with BCAA, Phe, Glu, creatine	0.0	0.0	0	0.0	0	0.0	0
TOTAL	336.0	28.0	33	56.0	67	0.0	0

)) *Second Meal after Workout*

	CALORIES	PROTEIN	%	CARBS	%	FAT	%
200 grams lean meat (raw weight)	155.1	34.6	89	0.0	0	1.9	11
Large garden salad	65.0	4.0	25	10.0	62	1.0	14
1 serving fruit	93.0	1.0	4	20.0	86	1.0	10
50 grams wild rice, raw	193.0	8.0	17	38.0	79	1.0	5
2 fish oil capsules	18.0	0.0	0	0.0	0	2.0	100
TOTAL	524.1	47.6	36	68.0	52	6.9	12

)) *Pre-Bed Meal*

	CALORIES	PROTEIN	%	CARBS	%	FAT	%
250 ml egg white	108.0	25.0	93	2.0	7	0.0	0
1 serving fruit	93.0	1.0	4	20.0	86	1.0	10
50 grams oats (raw)	187.0	8.0	17	32.0	68	3.0	14
TOTAL	201.0	34.0	68	54.0	107	4.0	18
GRAND TOTAL	4135.4	372.8	36	396.0	38	138.6	30

Nutrition for Nontraining Days (4 times per week):

)) First Breakfast Meal

ITEM	CALORIES	PROTEIN	%	CARBS	%	FAT	%
250 ml egg white	108.0	25.0	93	2.0	7	0.0	0
2 whole omega-3 eggs	137.0	13.0	38	1.0	3	9.0	59
1/4 cup mixed beans (kidney, etc.)	52.0	3.0	23	10.0	77	0.0	0
1 cup mixed vegetables	44.0	1.0	9	10.0	91	0.0	0
50 grams cashews	320.0	12.0	15	14.0	18	24.0	68
2 fish oil capsules	18.0	0.0	0	0.0	0	2.0	100
TOTAL	679.0	54.0	32	37.0	22	35.0	46

)) Second Breakfast Meal

ITEM	CALORIES	PROTEIN	%	CARBS	%	FAT	%
400 grams plain yogurt	249.0	14.0	22	19.0	31	13.0	47
50 grams almonds	322.0	12.0	15	10.0	12	26.0	73
2 scoops milk protein blend	212.0	40.0	75	4.0	8	4.0	17
TOTAL	783.0	66.0	34	33.0	17	43.0	49

)) First Lunch Meal

ITEM	CALORIES	PROTEIN	%	CARBS	%	FAT	%
200 grams lean meat (raw weight)	155.1	34.6	89	0.0	0	1.9	11
Large garden salad	65.0	4.0	25	10.0	62	1.0	14
1 teaspoon flax oil	45.0	0.0	0	0.0	0	5.0	100
1 teaspoon olive oil	45.0	0.0	0	0.0	0	5.0	100
50 grams cheese	126.0	6.0	19	12.0	38	6.0	43
2 fish oil capsules	18.0	0.0	0	0.0	0	2.0	100
TOTAL	454.1	44.6	39	22.0	19	20.9	41

)) Second Lunch Meal

ITEM	CALORIES	PROTEIN	%	CARBS	%	FAT	%
200 grams lean meat (raw weight)	155.1	34.6	89	0.0	0	1.9	11
Large garden salad	65.0	4.0	25	10.0	62	1.0	14
1 teaspoon flax oil	45.0	0.0	0	0.0	0	5.0	100
1 teaspoon olive oil	45.0	0.0	0	0.0	0	5.0	100
50 grams walnuts	176	4.0	9	4.0	9	16.0	82
TOTAL	486.1	42.6	35	14.0	12	28.9	53

)) *Dinner Meal*

ITEM	CALORIES	PROTEIN	%	CARBS	%	FAT	%
200 grams lean meat (raw weight)	155.1	34.6	89	0.0	0	1.9	11
Large garden salad	65.0	4.0	25	10.0	62	1.0	14
1 serving fruit	93.0	1.0	4	20.0	86	1.0	10
25 grams cashews	329.0	12.0	15	14.0	17	25.0	68
2 fish oil capsules	18.0	0.0	0	0.0	0	2.0	100
TOTAL	660.1	51.6	31	44.0	27	30.9	42

)) *Pre-Bed Meal*

ITEM	CALORIES	PROTEIN	%	CARBS	%	FAT	%
250 ml egg white	108.0	25.0	93	2.0	7	0.0	0
2 whole omega-3 eggs	137.0	13.0	38	1.0	3	9.0	59
1 serving fruit	93.0	1.0	4	20.0	86	1.0	10
50 grams cheese	126.0	6.0	19	12.0	38	6.0	43
TOTAL	338.0	45.0	53	35.0	41	16.0	43
GRAND TOTAL	3400.4	303.8	36	185.0	22	174.6	46

Because you'll continue to gain weight, you'll probably have to keep increasing energy intake as follows to keep the gains coming:

Week 1: As listed above

Week 2: Add ¼ cup mixed beans and 1 piece fruit to the first breakfast meal.

Week 3: Add 1 tablespoon peanut butter during second breakfast meal.

Week 4: Add 100 grams yam to dinner meal.

MENU #3 — PHASES III AND IV: STRENGTH PHASE AND HYPERTROPHY PHASE

In these final two phases, your actual plan will be similar to the last week of the previous phase. This should be enough to keep the gains coming. However, the meal plan does not have to remain constant throughout. If you're not growing, use the Decision-Making Matrix on page 182.

Nutrition for Training Days
(3 times per week for Phase III and 4 times per week for Phase IV)

》 First Breakfast Meal

ITEM	CALORIES	PROTEIN	%	CARBS	%	FAT	%
250 ml egg white	108.0	25.0	93	2.0	7	0.0	0
2 whole omega-3 eggs	137.0	13.0	38	1.0	3	9.0	59
1/2 cup mixed beans (kidney, etc.)	104.0	6.0	23	20.0	77	0.0	0
1 cup mixed vegetables	44.0	1.0	9	10.0	91	0.0	0
50 grams cashews	320.0	12.0	15	14.0	18	24.0	68
1 serving fruit	93.0	1.0	4	20.0	86	1.0	10
2 fish oil capsules	18.0	0.0	0	0.0	0	2.0	100
TOTAL	824.0	58.0	28	67.0	33	36.0	39

》 Second Breakfast Meal

ITEM	CALORIES	PROTEIN	%	CARBS	%	FAT	%
400 grams plain yogurt	249.0	14.0	22	19.0	31	13.0	47
50 grams almonds	322.0	12.0	15	10.0	12	26.0	73
1 tablespoon peanut butter	238.0	12.0	20	25.0	42	10.0	38
2 scoops milk protein blend	212.0	40.0	75	4.0	8	4.0	17
TOTAL	1021.0	78.0	31	58.0	23	53.0	47

》 First Lunch Meal

ITEM	CALORIES	PROTEIN	%	CARBS	%	FAT	%
200 grams lean meat (raw weight)	155.1	34.6	89	0.0	0	1.9	11
Large garden salad	65.0	4.0	25	10.0	62	1.0	14
1 teaspoon flax oil	45.0	0.0	0	0.0	0	5.0	100
1 teaspoon olive oil	45.0	0.0	0	0.0	0	5.0	100
50 grams cheese	126.0	6.0	19	12.0	38	6.0	43
2 fish oil capsules	18.0	0.0	0	0.0	0	2.0	100
TOTAL	454.1	44.6	39	22.0	19	20.9	41

MENU #3—*Continued*

)) Second Lunch Meal

ITEM	CALORIES	PROTEIN	%	CARBS	%	FAT	%
200 grams lean meat (raw weight)	155.1	34.6	89	0.0	0	1.9	11
Large garden salad	65.0	4.0	25	10.0	62	1.0	14
1 teaspoon flax oil	45.0	0.0	0	0.0	0	5.0	100
1 teaspoon olive oil	45.0	0.0	0	0.0	0	5.0	100
50 grams walnuts	176	4.0	9	4.0	9	16.0	82
TOTAL	486.1	42.6	35	14.0	12	28.9	53

)) Immediately before Workout

ITEM	CALORIES	PROTEIN	%	CARBS	%	FAT	%
1 serving recovery drink	336.0	28.0	33	56.0	67	0.0	0
with BCAA, Phe, Glu	0.0	0.0	0	0.0	0	0.0	0
TOTAL	336.0	28.0	33	56.0	67	0.0	0

)) Sip during Workout

ITEM	CALORIES	PROTEIN	%	CARBS	%	FAT	%
1 serving recovery drink	336.0	28.0	33	56.0	67	0.0	0
with BCAA, Phe, Glu	0.0	0.0	0	0.0	0	0.0	0
TOTAL	336.0	28.0	33	56.0	67	0.0	0

)) Immediately after Workout

ITEM	CALORIES	PROTEIN	%	CARBS	%	FAT	%
1 serving recovery drink	336.0	28.0	33	56.0	67	0.0	0
with BCAA, Phe, Glu, creatine	0.0	0.0	0	0.0	0	0.0	0
TOTAL	336.0	28.0	33	56.0	67	0.0	0

)) Second Meal after Workout

ITEM	CALORIES	PROTEIN	%	CARBS	%	FAT	%
200 grams lean meat (raw weight)	155.1	34.6	89	0.0	0	1.9	11
Large garden salad	65.0	4.0	25	10.0	62	1.0	14
1 serving fruit	93.0	1.0	4	20.0	86	1.0	10
50 grams wild rice raw	193.0	8.0	17	38.0	79	1.0	5
100 grams yam	128.0	2.0	6	30.0	94	0.0	0
2 fish oil capsules	18.0	0.0	0	0.0	0	2.0	100
TOTAL	652.1	49.6	30	98.0	60	6.9	9

)) Pre-Bed Meal

ITEM	CALORIES	PROTEIN	%	CARBS	%	FAT	%
250 ml egg white	108.0	25.0	93	2.0	7	0.0	0
1 serving fruit	93.0	1.0	4	20.0	86	1.0	10
50 grams oats (raw)	187.0	8.0	17	32.0	68	3.0	14
TOTAL	201.0	34.0	68	54.0	107	4.0	18
GRAND TOTAL	4646.4	390.8	34	481.0	41	149.6	29

Nutrition for Nontraining Days
(4 times per week for Phase III, 3 times per week for Phase IV)

⟫ First Breakfast Meal

ITEM	CALORIES	PROTEIN	%	CARBS	%	FAT	%
250 ml egg white	108.0	25.0	93	2.0	7	0.0	0
2 whole omega-3 eggs	137.0	13.0	38	1.0	3	9.0	59
½ cup mixed beans (kidney, etc.)	104.0	6.0	23	20.0	77	0.0	0
1 cup mixed vegetables	44.0	1.0	9	10.0	91	0.0	0
50 grams cashews	320.0	12.0	15	14.0	18	24.0	68
1 serving fruit	93.0	1.0	4	20.0	86	1.0	10
2 fish oil capsules	18.0	0.0	0	0.0	0	2.0	100
TOTAL	**824.0**	**58.0**	**28**	**67.0**	**33**	**36.0**	**39**

⟫ Second Breakfast Meal

ITEM	CALORIES	PROTEIN	%	CARBS	%	FAT	%
400 grams plain yogurt	249.0	14.0	22	19.0	31	13.0	47
50 grams almonds	322.0	12.0	15	10.0	12	26.0	73
1 tablespoon peanut butter	238.0	12.0	20	25.0	42	10.0	38
2 scoops milk protein blend	212.0	40.0	75	4.0	8	4.0	17
TOTAL	**1021.0**	**78.0**	**31**	**58.0**	**23**	**53.0**	**47**

⟫ First Lunch Meal

ITEM	CALORIES	PROTEIN	%	CARBS	%	FAT	%
200 grams lean meat (raw weight)	155.1	34.6	89	0.0	0	1.9	11
Large garden salad	65.0	4.0	25	10.0	62	1.0	14
1 teaspoon flax oil	45.0	0.0	0	0.0	0	5.0	100
1 teaspoon olive oil	45.0	0.0	0	0.0	0	5.0	100
50 grams cheese	126.0	6.0	19	12.0	38	6.0	43
2 fish oil capsules	18.0	0.0	0	0.0	0	2.0	100
TOTAL	**454.1**	**44.6**	**39**	**22.0**	**19**	**20.9**	**41**

⟫ Second Lunch Meal

ITEM	CALORIES	PROTEIN	%	CARBS	%	FAT	%
200 grams lean meat (raw weight)	155.1	34.6	89	0.0	0	1.9	11
Large garden salad	65.0	4.0	25	10.0	62	1.0	14
1 teaspoon flax oil	45.0	0.0	0	0.0	0	5.0	100
1 teaspoon olive oil	45.0	0.0	0	0.0	0	5.0	100
50 grams walnuts	176	4.0	9	4.0	9	16.0	82
TOTAL	**486.1**	**42.6**	**35**	**14.0**	**12**	**28.9**	**53**

MENU #3—*Continued*

)) *Dinner Meal*

ITEM	CALORIES	PROTEIN	%	CARBS	%	FAT	%
200 grams lean meat (raw weight)	155.1	34.6	89	0.0	0	1.9	11
Large garden salad	65.0	4.0	25	10.0	62	1.0	14
1 serving fruit	93.0	1.0	4	20.0	86	1.0	10
25 grams cashews	329.0	12.0	15	14.0	17	25.0	68
100 grams yam	128.0	2.0	6	30.0	94	0.0	0
2 fish oil capsules	18.0	0.0	0	0.0	0	2.0	100
TOTAL	788.1	53.6	27	74.0	38	30.9	35

)) *Pre-Bed Meal*

ITEM	CALORIES	PROTEIN	%	CARBS	%	FAT	%
250 ml egg white	108.0	25.0	93	2.0	7	0.0	0
2 whole omega-3 eggs	137.0	13.0	38	1.0	3	9.0	59
1 serving fruit	93.0	1.0	4	20.0	86	1.0	10
50 grams cheese	126.0	6.0	19	12.0	38	6.0	43
TOTAL	338.0	45.0	53	35.0	41	16.0	43
GRAND TOTAL	3911.4	321.8	33	270.0	28	185.6	43

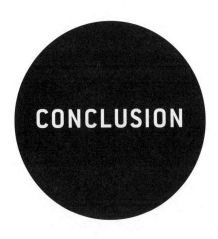

CONCLUSION

ANTICIPATING THE LONG ROAD AHEAD

>> By now, you should have a completely different perspective of what it takes to build muscle. In this book, you've learned all about the biomechanical and metabolic differences that set you apart from others around you. You've gained new insights into how to shop for, prepare, and even consume the types and amounts of food that you need to put on some size. Along the way, you've also probably developed a newfound respect for things such as the importance of workout nutrition, the need to train for strength, and even how improved flexibility can lead to dramatic improvements in the way your body functions. We've even provided you with a comprehensive step-by-step training program and sample menus to get you started on the road to your new physique. The only thing we didn't do is supply you with a plan for going forward. Or did we?

Unlike other training books, it should be fairly obvious by now that ours is not a "here, do this" sort of guide. Our objective when we set out wasn't to create some "quick fix" program for skinny guys looking to put on muscle mass. If you've been reading carefully up to this point, you know that just isn't possible. Any effective program causes physical change. If we design an optimal program for your body today, 3 months from now, you'll have a different body that needs a new program. So rather than just giving you one program for today and sending you on your merry way, our intention is to help you understand where your challenges lie and help you take the proper steps in addressing them. In that regard, this book very much embodies this notion: "Give a man a fish, and feed him for a day; teach him to fish, and feed him for a lifetime."

By reading this book once, twice, maybe even three times and understanding all the interesting anatomy and physiology, you'll be able to put the principles we've laid out into action. In doing so, you'll have a plan for how to eat and lift for many years to come. After all, we taught you how to correct common muscular imbalances (Chapter 6), we taught you proper program design variables (Chapter 4), and we taught you how to use an outcome-based nutritional strategy (Chapter 13). And the best part is that you'll do it in a healthy, well-rounded fashion. The inclusion of cardiovascular training, the heavy emphasis on fruits, vegetables, and fiber in your diet, and the attention paid to addressing your current physical liabilities make this far from just an exercise in vanity.

Don't Sweat the Small Stuff

At this point, you should have already begun the program or are getting ready to. In doing so, we have to ask a favor. In order for you to have the wherewithal to get through this program, you're not only going to have to understand our programs; you're going to have to put your trust in us. We've produced astounding results in trainees across the world with programs similar to those contained in this book. Therefore, we respectfully ask that you stick with us throughout the full four-phase program. In doing so, refrain from making little alterations to the program as you go along, regardless of what your gym mates think or suggest.

Throwing in a couple of extra sets of arm work or increasing the frequency and/or duration of the cardiovascular work is a no-no. Doing a few extra sets of benches or squats; again, a no-no. We know some of you may feel like you "need it," but trust us; you

GOING FORWARD

But what about after you've reached your goal? Let's say for instance that you follow the program to a tee and end up adding an impressive amount to muscle to your frame. What then? Should you still steer clear of treadmills and biceps curls at all costs? And what about eating? Do you keep packing it away like you've got a hollow leg or is it alright to eat more like a normal human being? While you may not have to be quite as extreme as you do throughout the duration of the program, you will have to adhere to most of the principles we've set forth in this book to some degree. Don't worry though, we've provided you with a handy maintenance guide below.

>> Be sure to regularly adjust your caloric intake to reflect changes in your physique by using the Decision-Making Matrix (page 182). Whether you want to shed body fat or continue to bulk up, don't do it in a haphazard manner.

>> Once you've reached your desired weight and percent body fat, continue to employ nutrient partitioning to help maintain the gains you've made. Don't think it's safe to go back to your old bad habits! Continuing to eat the same good foods, simply adjust your energy intake in such a way as to maintain, gain, or lose according to your immediate goals.

>> When training, whether you design your own workouts or follow a "premade" routine from a book or magazine, make sure you keep the focus on heavy, compound lifts.

>> As your training experience grows, so too will your capacity to handle a slightly larger training volume. Just be sure that the volume increase is primarily in the form of multiple-set, low-rep work and not the standard bodybuilding approach (i.e., 8 sets of 3 versus 3 sets of 8).

>> During intensive muscle-building phases, keep the cardio and any other extraneous physical activity (pick-up basketball, swimming, etc.) to a minimum. You can always enjoy that stuff during off weeks from training; just be sure to eat enough to support the additional activity.

>> Speaking of off weeks, we recommend taking a full 7 days off from structured lifting at least two or three times a year to allow your body to regenerate a bit. One full week of active rest should follow the program contained in this book.

>> When trying to strip off body fat and fine-tune your physique, increasing the frequency of your cardio up to 3 or 4 times per week is permissible; just try to stay away from long, drawn-out workouts. Brief, intense bouts of exercise that are far removed from your strength training are your best bets.

don't. All you'll be doing is putting a greater strain on your recuperative abilities and impeding your progress. Besides, if you feel like you still have the energy to do a few sets of curls or some extra crunches at the end of your workouts, you didn't work anywhere near hard enough on your compound lifts!

As for the cardio, allow us to let you in on a little secret: Not all of the weight you gain on this program is going to be muscle. Unfortunately, it simply isn't possible to make large increases in muscle mass without picking up a little extra body fat along the way. Not a lot, mind you, but enough to obscure those abs a bit and make some of your veins a little less visible. For some of you, this won't be a big deal because any increase in weight will likely be a welcome sight. For others, though, a little extra fat will send you frantically running for the treadmill or elliptical machine. Don't do it! The objective during this period is to gain some much-needed size; there'll be plenty of time later on to shave off any excess fat and show off your new physique. Who cares if your abs are a little less visible for a while? It's no big deal for a scrawny guy to sport a six-pack anyway. But add another 15 or 20 pounds to your frame, and that same six-pack will definitely turn a few heads.

You might also be wondering why you're not training smaller muscle groups such as your calves and forearms. Admittedly, the program isn't exactly chock-full of wrist curls and heel raises. That isn't because we forgot to put them in; we designed the program this way for a reason. Remember back in Chapter 2 where we talked about treating your body as an entire organism and not just a conglomeration of different muscle groups? Consuming enough calories and focusing on heavy, compound lifts will make the entire organism grow. Don't waste your time chasing after these smaller muscle groups. Your calves will get called into play on exercises such as hang cleans and negative leg curls, and your forearms will be working like crazy during deadlifts and pullups. Ask yourself for a second, what do you think will add more mass to those forearms, 20-rep sets of wrist curls, or deadlifting twice your body weight without the aid of lifting straps? Starting to get the idea?

The Next Step

At this point, we've done everything we can do with a book. However, so as not to leave you hanging, we've developed a fully interactive Web site (www.scrawnytobrawny.com) that's available to support you through your 16-week Scrawny to Brawny transformation and beyond.

The next 16 weeks are pretty simple, and your plate will be full (both literally and figuratively). Get ready to do an awful lot of lifting, whether it involves heavy barbells or yet another forkful into your perpetually open trap. And if you want to share stories, successes, or recipes with other scrawny guys on their path to bulking up, pop over to our Web site. The site will be set up so that you can ask questions about your own personal programs, about your own nutritional plans, or about anything else that pops into your mind. What a tremendous asset it is to join with training brothers and sisters from around the world striving to transform their own physique challenges from roadblocks into speed bumps.

And once your 16-week program is up, and you're ready to move on, revisit this book or the site for program design tips, exercise selections, new recipes, or just a little support for your upcoming stage. After all, by the end of your 16-week transformation, you'll be bigger, stronger, and most important, better educated about training and nutrition than you ever have before. You'll no longer be that poor slob who busts his butt in the gym with nothing to show for his efforts. No more mindlessly going from one program to the next, searching for "the one." No more randomly guessing about the amounts and types of foods you should be eating. From here on in, you're in control of your own physical destiny. This book provides the plan; you provide the action. And so, for one last time, what are you waiting for, *Skinny?* Get to work!

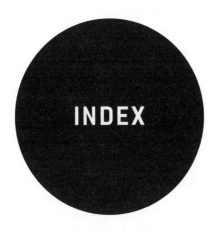

INDEX

Boldface page references indicate photographs. Underscored references indicate boxed text.